jailhouse Too

A TRIBUTE TO MY COLLEAGUES

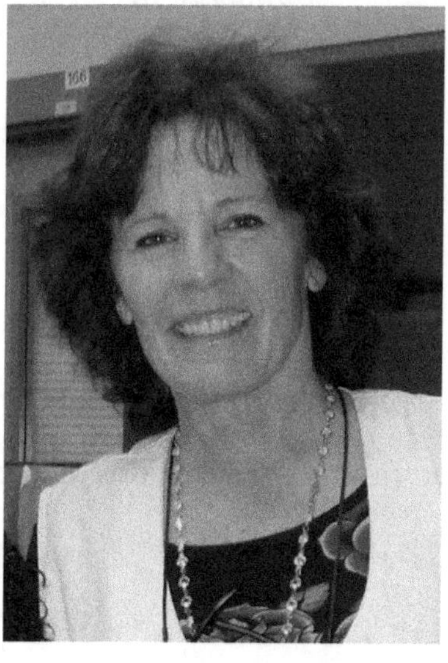

Nancy Smith, RN

Jailhouse is a work of nonfiction.

Names and identifying details have been changed.

Library of Congress Cataloging-in-Publication Data

Smith, Nancy

Jailhouse / by Nancy Smith

Includes index.

ISBN: 979-8-9970677-1-7

Printed in the United States of America

Praise for Jailhouse Too

Insightful

It takes a special person to practice nursing. Nurses must jump into the lives of their patients at a rough point. Yet many nurses find their calling in this unusual health care setting.

Astonishing

If I were an inmate needing medical care, I'd want Nancy to be my nurse

Well Written

It is not just a good read. It is one of "those books" that stays on your desk and bookcase- - - not as a "how-to book", but for insight into compassionate care.

Wonderful

These stories reveal compassion from a real-world perspective.

Fascinating

Based on her real experiences, Nancy journeys beyond jail walls to share a nurse's unimaginable and shocking revelations of events, behaviors, and relationships in a county jail.

Unique

These books are a must-have for anyone interested in creating a compassionate correctional health service.

Reflective

Compassion has become a prominent issue in health policy and practice in recent years, with numerous "failures" in nursing care receiving media coverage. These stories reveal a range of issues that must be addressed - including leadership and organizational culture.

Marvelous

These books describe "real" nursing as many incarcerated patients need health teaching, self-care skills, and chronic disease management.

Good Read

These books were very enlightening about compassionate medical care in jail.

Thoughtful

Is correctional nursing for you? The pages of these insightful books may provide answers.

Contents

Jailhouse Too

The people I admire most in the corrections setting are those who make a significant positive impact every day.

The people I admire most in the corrections setting are not the ones whose names appear in headlines. They are not famous. They are not praised publicly. Most days, no one outside the walls even knows they exist. Yet every single day, they step into a place most people fear, bringing with them skill, steadiness, and heart. They show up—in chaos, in crisis, in suffering—and they make a difference that rarely gets noticed. This book is for them.

In Jailhouse—Book One—I introduced myself: Nurse Nancy Smith. I traced the long, winding road of my nursing career—why I chose this profession, how I was drawn into correctional nursing, and what daily life looked like inside Oakwood Correctional Facility. I described the rhythm of the medical unit, the relentless pace of the charge nurse, and a major task force effort to improve communication and care. The stories centered largely on the inmates—their illnesses, their humanity, their struggles—and the challenge of delivering compassionate healthcare in a place designed for punishment, not healing.

Jailhouse Too—Book Two—turns the lens outward.

In this book, the stories focus on the people who stand shoulder-to-shoulder inside these walls: doctors, nurses, deputies, mental health professionals, and the support staff who hold the system together. I write about those whose quiet competence and can-do attitude made the impossible feel manageable—and yes, about a few whose presence made every shift harder. This is an honest telling. A human one. I also write about something close to my heart: the Oakwood feral cat program. Even in a place built of concrete and steel, compassion finds its way in. Caring for those animals reminded me—again and again—that tenderness can survive anywhere, even behind razor wire.

Truth be told, I never imagined my nursing journey would end here.

After decades of nursing—walking polished hospital corridors, racing through acute care units, sitting in silence with families during hospice goodbyes, and offering dignity in homes where life was fading—I found myself somewhere I never expected to be. Behind locked gates. Steel doors. Razor wire. Rules that never bend. A jail.

Correctional nursing is not just another specialty. It is a calling forged at the collision point between chaos and compassion. It is far more than passing medications or checking vital signs. It is about delivering ethical, humane healthcare to one of the most marginalized populations in our society. When someone becomes incarcerated, their need for healthcare does not vanish. For many, it finally begins.

People arrive carrying years—sometimes lifetimes—of neglect. Uncontrolled diabetes. Dangerous blood pressure. Infected wounds. Rotted teeth. Untreated mental illness. Addiction. Trauma layered upon trauma. These are not just diagnoses; they are the echoes of lives lived without access, stability, or mercy. Pain does not pause because someone is wearing orange. Withdrawal is merciless. Mental anguish is relentless. And sometimes, the first moment of kindness an inmate receives comes when a nurse calls their name and looks them in the eye.

Before Oakwood, I had already seen hardship. I had sat beside lonely veterans in VA hospitals. I had held hands in hospice rooms when words had run out. I had managed crises over the phone in the dead of night. Once, in a patient's crumbling home, I calmly reviewed medications while sitting on newspaper on a filthy couch—as a foot-long rat ran along the wall beside me.

I also had uplifting experiences of caring for the aged parents of several Hollywood celebrities. Their homes were adorned with classic movie memorabilia. One housed an Oscar.

Still, nothing quite prepared me for jail.

I've witnessed high-adrenaline emergencies—cell extractions, medical crises, psychiatric breakdowns—but this book is not about shock value. It is a tribute to the good people who show up every day inside those walls. The medical staff. The deputies. The mental health professionals. The quiet heroes who make a difference where few are willing to look.

Under the protection of sheriff's deputies, I once knelt beside an inmate whose face had been slashed in retaliation—blood pooling at his feet. Deputies formed a silent circle of safety around me. Medical staff moved with practiced urgency. No one flinched. No one turned away. That moment—like so many others—taught me what correctional healthcare truly is: unpredictable, intense, dangerous at times, and profoundly human.

What struck me most after years inside Oakwood was this: the public has no idea what truly happens behind those walls.

Correctional healthcare is invisible. What people think they know about it comes from sensational headlines and television dramas—violence, lockdowns, gangs. That is only a fraction of the truth. What's missing are the quiet moments. The teamwork. The compassion. The deputy who wipes blood from a man's face. The nurse who refuses to give up on a patient that everyone else has written off. The mental health counselor who patiently talks someone back from the edge.

These people became my family inside the walls. This book is their story. I had to write it—true stories, snapshots of life behind bars. Some are intense. Some are tender. All are real.

These pages shine a light on the deeply human connections that can exist between inmates, nurses, doctors, mental health professionals, deputies, chaplains, and administrators. Yes, there are crises—but often there are moments of connection. Unexpected laughter. A hand on a shoulder. A drawing slipped through a food slot. A deputy standing watch so care can happen safely.

This is not a traditional memoir. There is no single protagonist. Instead, there are windows—each offering a glimpse into a world that is complex, chaotic, heartbreaking, and unexpectedly full of grace. Terrible things happen in jail. But so do acts of kindness. So does healing. So does humanity. And that is what I want you to see.

Oakwood Correctional Facility

Oakwood evolved from a 19th-century almshouse to a modern jail with complex housing structures, custody levels, and rising violence. Not just a building; it was a living organism—breathing tension, pulsing with unpredictability. Working among the mentally ill, the broken, the angry, and the forgotten forced me to confront parts of myself I hadn't known existed. It pushed me to understand how tightly operations, safety, and healthcare intertwine. I had to grow stronger, gentler, braver. Its walls held the ghosts of its history and the weight of thousands of lives passing through it. I learned the rhythms of each housing area, the unspoken rules, the way violence could erupt from silence.

As of today, Oakwood Correctional Facility has expanded into a primary county detention center that houses about 2,100 male and 500 female inmates on any given day. Men and women are housed in separate buildings, and there are separate wings with capabilities for medium- and minimum-security prisoners. Minimum security inmates are housed dormitory-style, complete with bunk beds. Oakwood employs approximately 300 County Department of Corrections (Office of the Sheriff) officers and 25 administrative support staff.

Oakwood Medical

Inmates can interact with professional staff every day; nurses and mental health staff are available 24 hours/day. They see MDs at medical appointments Monday through Friday. Registered nurses see inmates (patients) daily at sick call, detox checks, lab draws, and diabetic call (checking blood sugar values 2-4 times/day), as well as for wound care, monitoring high blood pressure, and after "man-downs" for medical clearance. Man-downs occur with altercations, accidents, ingestion of drugs, suicide attempts, hunger strikes, c/o chest pain, pregnant women in labor, and escape attempts. Inmates also have appointments with dentists, orthopedic PA, psychiatrists, psychologists, and therapists in the Medical Dept.

Healthcare in jail is like practicing medicine in a storm. People arrive shattered—detoxing, broken, terrified, sick, untreated for years. Intake screening can feel like a triage battlefield; detox can feel like watching someone unravel from the inside. Chronic illness, psychiatric crises, emergency after emergency—nothing at Oakwood resembled hospital work. I had to learn to trust my instincts, move fast, adapt constantly, think in both clinical and security terms, and see the human being beneath the charges.

Medical, dental, and mental health services are integral to the care provided at Oakwood. Each inmate undergoes a medical screening (interview by an RN) at the time of booking. The information gathered is confidentially protected by the Medical unit to ensure appropriate care.

Funding and resource allocation impact the quality of care. Affordability, staffing shortages, and treatment delays are continuing challenges. Prisoners face numerous health issues, often impacted by limited preventive care and overcrowding/understaffing. Chronic illnesses, mental health disorders, and emergency medical services are among the most pressing concerns.

Typical Experiences As Charge Nurse

I walk into the jail on a late October afternoon wearing my favorite Halloween scrubs—horns and a halo stitched onto fabric in what feels like a quiet act of defiance. The inmates smile. For a moment, there is lightness. But it never lasts long. The shift begins with report, and already I feel the weight settle in: detoxing bodies, unstable blood sugars, fragile minds, people hanging in the balance while the clock keeps moving.

Once report ends, the chaos blooms instantly. Diabetic call. Lobby filling. Phones ringing without mercy. Lab values come in dangerous and urgent. Doctors call. Family members call, voices tight with fear. Staff call out sick. I am constantly scanning—doorways, hands, objects—because my safety is as much a part of my job as my compassion. Forty inmates can be waiting at once, and somehow we are expected to keep everyone safe, alive, and seen.

Then the radio crackles. "Man-down."

The words slice through everything. My heart spikes before my mind catches up. Lockdown is ordered. Appointments stop mid-sentence. I grab the crash cart, oxygen tanks, AED, medications, laptop—everything that might mean the difference between life and death. I don't yet know what I'm walking into, only that time is already slipping away.

As we move quickly through the facility, inmates step aside. Some even help us carry equipment up the stairs. In a place built on punishment, I still find humanity showing up when it matters most. That never stops surprising me.

When I reach him, he's face down on the ground, seizing violently. Unresponsive. The scene sharpens into pure focus. We lay him on a clean pad, start an IV, tend to his wounds. The deputies call for a Code 3. Sirens are coming. I piece together his history—new booking, no reported alcohol use this time, but old records tell the truth. Withdrawal. His body is paying the price.

The fire department arrives and administers IV Ativan. The seizure finally breaks. They rush him out, and just like that, the emergency leaves with them. We don't get closure. We don't get relief. We walk back to Medical because the work never pauses long enough for that.

Phones are still ringing. Inmates are still waiting. Paperwork is still piling up. I eat my lunch in minutes, barely tasting it, and dive back into documentation—charting the man-down, calling the ER, recording vitals, making sure nothing gets missed, even though everything feels overwhelming.

Then I answer a phone call that cracks me open. It's a mother. She didn't know where her son was for days. Now she knows he's in jail. She is frantic, sobbing, desperate for reassurance. I can't give her medical details—he refused to sign a release—but I hear the terror in her voice. I tell her the deputies are watching him. I promise to involve mental health. I try to steady her with my voice while my chest tightens. When the call ends, I sit there, stunned by how heavy her grief feels in my hands. I pass the information to mental health, trusting they will follow through. But the tears she cried stay with me. I take that call home with me. I always do.

As the shift winds down, nothing actually slows. Phones ring until the last minute. The report must be given. Crises blur into routine. I am exhausted in a way that sinks deep into my bones—but I am also reminded why this work matters. In this place, I witness fear, kindness, desperation, resilience, and love in their rawest forms.

I can't control how long a life lasts. But every shift like this reminds me that I can help widen it—just a little—by showing up fully, even when it hurts.

Adult Custody Health Services Task Force

A few years into my work at Oakwood, I began to feel something was wrong—not loudly wrong, but persistently, painfully off. Complaints were coming from everywhere. Nurses. Doctors. Mental health. Clerical staff. Janitorial. Different voices, same exhaustion. People were frustrated, worn down, and unheard. What troubled me most wasn't the complaints themselves—it was the silence afterward. There was nowhere for those concerns to land. No path forward. Just people carrying their frustration back to the floor shift after shift.

I remember sitting in a leadership meeting one morning, the air heavy with fatigue, when our Medical Director, Dr. Alex Sherbakov, finally said what we were all thinking. He looked around the room and said, *"We're all hearing the same problems—but from different angles. What if we stopped working in silos and actually came together?"*

Something stirred in me when he said that. Not a feeling of relief exactly—but possibility.

He spoke about creating a multidisciplinary Task Force. Not another committee that talked in circles, but a group with real voices—people who worked nights, people who cleaned floors, people who passed meds under pressure, people who answered phones and absorbed everyone else's stress.

When we held our first meeting, the room felt uncertain. Folding chairs. Someone brought a plate of fruit. Some drank strong coffee from a random assemblage of mugs that could have come from the Goodwill Store. People were sitting with guarded expressions, arms crossed, not sure if this was just another empty gesture. I could feel the skepticism in the air.

Greg asked bluntly, *"What exactly are we trying to do here?"*

I took a breath and said, *"We're trying to understand each other. And we're trying to fix things—together."*

That moment mattered. I could see it. The tension softened just a bit

As the meetings continued, stories began to spill out—things people had been carrying quietly for years. Maria talked about working nights and not knowing who was on call for mental health, and being afraid to wake the wrong person at 3 a.m. Tom spoke about trying to clean safely without knowing when areas were suddenly in use. Then Greg said something that stopped us all cold:

"We don't even know who people are anymore," he said. *"New faces come and go. We don't know names, or even who works here."*

It wasn't an operational issue—it was a human one. It hit me hard.

Someone suggested making posters. Faces. Names. Departments. Such a small thing. Almost embarrassingly simple. And yet, when those posters went up, the change was immediate. People started greeting each other by name. New staff felt welcomed instead of invisible. Long-timers felt recognized again. I watched connections quietly return in a place that had forgotten how to see itself.

As the Task Force grew, so did our courage. One day Dr. Sherbakov said, *"We solve problems together—but we don't have a shared foundation. Let's define who we are."* So we did. Slowly. Carefully. Highlighting Respect. Accountability. Compassion. Collaboration. We argued over words, revised sentences, and weighed what truly mattered. When we finally signed that Vision and Mission statement—every one of us—I felt something rare in institutional work: pride.

<table>
<tr><th colspan="2">ADULT CUSTODY HEALTH SERVICES</th></tr>
<tr><th>MISSION</th><th>CORE VALUES</th></tr>
<tr><td>As an integral part of County Health, we work in partnership with other departments to meet the complex, challenging healthcare needs of patients residing in Adult Custody facilities, focusing on health promotion, disease prevention, and management of acute and chronic conditions.

We contribute to the general public's well-being through health education, prevention, surveillance, and treatment of communicable diseases, taking care of underserved populations and raising awareness of a variety of public health issues.</td><td>Patient care with compassion, empathy, respect, integrity, and pride

Staff: our most important resource

Teamwork: foundation of our success

Custody staff is part of our team

Streamline, re-evaluate, and continuously improve
- Work smarter, not harder</td></tr>
<tr><th colspan="2">VISION</th></tr>
<tr><td colspan="2">We operate as an integrated and empowered healthcare team by motivating, monitoring, and generously supporting one another, so that each team member reaches their full potential.

Our care exceeds regulatory and community standards, while being efficient and cost-effective. Care is rendered in a physical setting that accommodates patients' special needs.

Emphasis is on preventative care, patient education, rehabilitation, and discharge planning, which are provided with a goal of reducing recidivism.

We are nationally recognized for our excellence and leadership in the correctional health services field. We are a unique center of learning for healthcare professionals.</td></tr>
</table>

That Task Force didn't fix everything, but it changed something essential. It turned complaints into conversations. It replaced isolation with partnership. It reminded people that their voices mattered—whether they wore scrubs, carried keys, or pushed a mop. And it changed me, too. It deepened my belief that when people are truly heard—when they are respected and invited into the solution—real, lasting change isn't just possible. It's inevitable.

The following stories focus on the people who stand shoulder-to-shoulder inside those walls: doctors, nurses, deputies, mental health professionals, and the support staff who hold the system together.

Bonnie

Bonnie was a gifted mental-health clinician whose gentle humor and fierce compassion brought healing to countless inmates. She created trauma-recovery groups and listened without judgment in a place where listening was rare. Her struggle with electromagnetic hypersensitivity forced her early retirement, leaving a void that broke my heart. When she left, the building seemed to dim. We lost more than a coworker—we lost a healer.

There are countless stories about inmates interacting with professional staff in amazing, confusing, and extraordinary ways. Medical staff call inmates "patients," and Mental Health (MH) staff refer to them as "clients." Some staff respond with judgment or indifference. Others, like Bonnie, showed nothing but kindness and genuine empathy.

Bonnie stood out. Tall, blonde, striking, and in her fifties, she was an MH therapist at Oakwood Correctional Facility. But what really made her beautiful was the way she treated the inmates. She listened. She cared. When Bonnie met with someone, the line for MH visits magically disappeared for the rest of the day. That didn't happen with anyone else.

Inmates had an open opportunity to ask to speak with MH department staff. The inmate needed to give their unit deputy the reason they were requesting to see someone from MH: anxiety, not sleeping, worried about court/charges, and the most serious complaint – feeling suicidal.

A few staff members felt the inmates don't deserve the same level of care rendered to patients in clinics, hospitals, and home settings because...well...they are INMATES. But after Bonnie met with inmates, there were no more same-day follow-up requests for MH visits, as there were when other MH staff met with inmates. It was evident Bonnie's heart was in her work.

She also demonstrated her dedication to inmates by trying to get management to provide more services. Bonnie's efforts resulted in the creation of Trauma Recovery groups to help the inmates deal with things like childhood sexual abuse, physical and emotional abuse, and human trafficking. Her actions contributed to keeping the peace in the facility.

"You okay, Bonnie?" I asked one evening after a late shift. We were walking out together, which was unusual—I usually stayed behind to feed the feral cats.

She gave a half-smile. "Not really. I'm avoiding home. It's become... kind of a nightmare."

"What happened?" I asked.

She sighed and looked at the pavement. "It started a couple of weeks ago. I came home and felt this overwhelming, almost painful energy. Numbness, buzzing, like my whole body was being invaded. It was...awful."

I raised an eyebrow. "Energy?"

"Electromagnetic," she said. "I'm hypersensitive to it. My naturopaths confirmed it. Turns out, the new neighbors installed a 5G internet router. The most powerful one on the market."

"Oof."

"I tried talking to them," she continued. "The mom agreed to switch to a wired setup. I called the router company for instructions, and I bought all the materials.

But her daughter? She was glued to her iPad. Insisted it wouldn't work "wired."

"She's not wrong," I said. "iPads need wireless."

Bonnie nodded, defeated. "The mom caved. I had already painted one wall with special paint to block smart meter radiation. I even took the power company to court and won. They reimbursed me for the cost of the paint. But I couldn't do that with the wall next to their unit. The HOA manager suggested covering the walls with foil. Can you imagine living with foil on your walls? I tried putting foil on a small area of the wall – it looked really bad."

"Shiny. Very futuristic," I joked, trying to lighten the mood.

She chuckled weakly. "I made repeated trips next door. I pleaded with them to limit the screen time on their digital TVs, iPads, and cell phones. The daughter is a big gamer. The daughter even called the cops on me!

"The officer showed up, listened to the complaint, and said, 'You called me for this? You're wasting my time.' Then walked out, without writing a report.

"I started sleeping at the office," she went on. "It was the only place I didn't feel the effects. I have shielding clothes, but they're too heavy to wear. Finally, the neighbors agreed to turn off the router at 1 a.m. every night. I was going home after that."

"How the hell did you keep showing up here like everything was normal?"

"Because those inmates in there," she nodded back toward the jail, "need me to be present. I can't let my mess spill over into their healing."

I myself didn't sleep that night. But despite all of the problems at Bonnie's home, she was able to refocus and truly help people at work.

Later, Bonnie bought a 1997 VW Jetta – no electromagnetic parts in this vehicle. She got special permission from the Captain to bypass the metal detector because it gave her terrible headaches. Unfortunately, it was time-limited. When the exemption expired and wasn't renewed, she decided to retire.

As I said, her absence left a void. The inmates lost more than a therapist. They lost one of the few people who saw them as human beings.

According to the World Health Organization Fact Sheet 296, “Electromagnetic hypersensitivity, also known as EHS, is a condition in which people have a wide range of symptoms that they believe are caused by exposure to electromagnetic fields (EMFs). EHS has no convincing scientific basis and is not a recognized medical diagnosis.” Symptoms may include headaches, fatigue, difficulty concentrating, sleep disturbances, burning sensations, skin irritation, and dizziness. A 2001 survey (International Journal of Hygiene and Environmental Health) found that people self-diagnosing as having EHS related their symptoms most frequently to cell sites, followed by mobile phones, cordless phones, microwave ovens, fluorescent lights, and power lines.

> ***My teacher told me not to worry about***
> ***spelling because in the future***
> ***there will be autocorrect.***
> ***And for that I am eternally grapefruit.***
> - joke about AI spellcheck

I See Dead People

Oakwood whispered when the halls were quiet. Its long history and eerie atmosphere fed constant ghost stories—apparitions in cells, shadowy former coworkers, children crying in corners, even Native American spirits said to roam old construction sites near burial remains. Whether real or not, the stories revealed something deeper: the building held memory—grief, folklore, mystery, and the echoes of lives long gone.

In the 1870s, the acreage that would later become Oakwood was owned by a farmer who raised thoroughbred horses and built a Victorian mansion on the estate. The County bought the property for $24,000 in 1884 and began using it as an almshouse – a shelter for the elderly and impoverished, prompting residents to dub the mansion: the "palace for the poor." The site became a compassionate haven for the homeless to live and work on the farm, providing them with shelter and meaningful employment. In the 1950s, the County began using the almshouse to house low-risk prisoners, establishing what would become the Oakwood Correctional Complex. When area residents wanted to incorporate as a city, they faced a dilemma because the law required a minimum population of 500, but the town had only 400 residents. Oakwood had an equal-sized population. Through a creative solution, the County allowed the Oakwood inhabitants to be counted, which validated the incorporation in 1954.

Over the decades, many unusual stories have come out of Oakwood regarding sightings of ghosts and apparitions. Several corrections staff, civilians, and inmates have seen some weird things throughout the facility.

The Medical building in particular has been a hotspot for ghostly encounters. Night shift nurses working the 11 PM-7 AM rotation reported seeing a woman in a long, flowing white gown walking the back corridor. Veteran nurses with over two decades of experience recognized her as a former colleague who passed away years ago from cancer.

Inmates have also contributed to the facility's supernatural lore. Several female inmates saw a young female "ghost" crying in one of the bathroom stalls in one of the oldest buildings. No one knew who she was. I have not been able to find any history of female inmates dying in this building, but some inmates go as far as to claim that ghostly presences are scattered throughout the facility.

One of the most intriguing narratives involves Deputy Moroccomole, a veteran officer with a remarkable history of paranormal experiences. Since childhood, he perceived entities and spirits that no one else could see. He has had neighbors who have passed away come to him (he says they are standing next to him) to pass on messages to loved ones. He doesn't share his experiences with many coworkers. It's just not something to discuss casually.

A particularly compelling story involves the construction of Oakwood's final building in 1993. During such projects, deputies are assigned to construction sites on the facility to ensure inmates do not venture over and get hurt or remove equipment. At one point, workers digging in the soil discovered what appeared to be the burial remains of the native Indians who populated the territory in the 1800s. Construction was stopped, and archaeologists were summoned.

Deputy M was stationed near a locked tool shed as the archeologist studied the site when he witnessed a remarkable vision: a Native American in full traditional headdress, chanting and dancing beside the shed. Remarkably, the archaeologist remained completely unaware of this supernatural display. Deputy M soon realized he was the sole witness to this incredible spectacle.

The apparition vanished as quickly as it had appeared, leaving the deputy in awe.

Despite his extraordinary experiences, Deputy M was known for maintaining a cheerful disposition, a rare and remarkable trait in a correctional environment.

These stories of Oakwood blend historical facts with supernatural speculation, creating a complex saga that transcends traditional institutional history. While some may view these accounts with skepticism, they nonetheless contribute to Oakwood's unique cultural identity, transforming it in people's minds from a mere administrative facility to a place of intrigue, compassion, and unexplained phenomena.

> ***Do the best you can until you know better. Then, when you know better, do better.***
> \- Maya Angelou

Six Degrees of Separation

Oakwood reminded me how small the world is. I kept running into unlikely connections —a dental office manager's boyfriend, a former Jazzercise acquaintance, even a rescued Bengal cat adopted by a local auto dealership manager. Each one of these felt like a quiet wink from the universe, proof that our lives are braided in unseen ways.

It is amazing how synchronicities sometimes just happen to work their way into our lives. Synchronicity is a term coined by psychologist Carl Jung to describe the occurrence of events that are related, but not causal. In other words, these events do not have a logical explanation behind them. They just happen. But there is meaning behind them if you are willing to look for it.

I prepared for another exciting routine appointment with my dentist, Dr. Denny Martin. I had known him for a long time, and he knew I had worked as a nurse at Oakwood for over 15 years.

My dentist always had interesting stories to tell his patients...

For example, at previous appointments he'd regaled me with stories of being with work furlough inmates employed at the local auto manufacturing plant while he was working his way through college. He said that back in the day, they would return to Oakwood at night after having worked there all day.

At this appointment, Dr. Martin had an unusual request.

His wife, a dentist in another city, had hired an office manager she really liked.

Apparently, the office manager's boyfriend, Dustin, had gotten into trouble and was in jail at Oakwood. According to my dentist, this young man was a really good kid who'd made some bad choices. His parents had passed away when he was young, and Dustin was raised by his grandfather. After his grandfather passed away, he was left a large house and an inheritance.

Over the years, he found roommates to rent rooms in the house to make some money. One evening, he made the mistake of driving drunk and got arrested for a DUI and other charges. Dustin was at Oakwood waiting to go to court. Dr. Martin asked me if I could check on him.

I replied I would be happy to check on this young man.

My opportunity to speak with Dustin came the next week. I sent out an invitation to Medical – this piece of paper had the inmate's name, inmate number (PFN), housing info (Barracks and bunk), and reason for the invitation. I wrote on the invitation that I was requesting a medical check. I believe word got back to him that a nurse would be checking on him.

He walked into Medical, took a seat, and started looking around. I found the invitation he had given to the Medical deputy and called out his name. He raised his hand. I was surprised to see a very clean-cut, good-looking young man who had a bit of a "deer in the headlights" look.

I introduced myself and placed the blood pressure cuff on his arm (to go along with the request to see him for medical reasons).

I quietly explained that Dr. Martin had asked me to check on him. I asked him if I could help him with anything. He smiled and replied, "How long have you worked at Oakwood as a nurse?"

I told him.

He continued, "Then you must know Kathy Benson. She is my next-door neighbor!"

I was totally caught off guard (and civilian staff are always on guard at Oakwood).

Kathy had been my manager at Oakwood for several years before she retired, after which we hung out and became friends.

I laughed and laughed! I told him I knew Kathy. Once I came back to my senses and remembered why I had called him to Medical, I asked him one more time if I could help him with anything. He very politely declined my offer. I told him if he needed anything Medical, he could come back, but I might not be scheduled there that day. He thanked me. I thanked him.

I called Dr. Martin to tell him I had seen Dustin and about our interesting conversation. He thanked me for checking in on him. I also emailed Kathy and explained how I happened to meet her next-door neighbor at Oakwood! She explained that Dustin had had a difficult time losing his parents and then his grandfather. Kathy said his new girlfriend was a good influence on him. She said they were planning on getting married.

At my next appointment with Dr. Martin, he cheerfully related the details of how well the story had turned out for Dustin. He was released from Oakwood, and received fines and probation. Dustin was doing great and getting married soon. He had turned his life around and it looked like he would not be coming back to Oakwood.

Another time I was coming to work, I recognized Jean, a woman I had been with in a Jazzercize class in the 1990s. She was walking into Oakwood's entry. We recognized each other and quickly caught up.

Then I HAD to ask, "What the heck are you doing here?" She replied that she had been ticketed with a citation for not being correctly licensed for her massage therapy practice. She didn't have the money to pay, so she chose community service. While performing her community service, she inadvertently left behind a therapeutic shoe fashioned for a physical disability, to enable her to walk correctly. She was trying to find the Lost and Found section of Oakwood. I wished her well and continued on to work.

I also ran into schoolmates of my kids while working at Oakwood Medical. I had been an elementary school substitute teacher, so I knew a lot of the younger kids. A few turned up at Oakwood after they turned 18. I never asked questions, but they all looked rather sheepish as they said: “I didn’t know you worked here.”

At one point, I bought a new Prius from the Toyota dealership across the street from Oakwood. Purchasing a new vehicle is always accompanied by mandatory warranty follow-ups at specific intervals. I always felt out of place at car dealerships because I didn’t know much about cars.

When I began the warranty appointments, I would drop off the car before work and pick it up at my dinner break.

In an attempt to ease my anxiety about being in the dealership, I started telling the guys there about the kitties I fed at Oakwood at night. To my surprise, the staff began telling me about the cats that hung around the dealership during the day. It sounded like they saw some of the same kitties I fed at night.

Around this time, I noticed a new stray cat who had wandered into the area where I fed the Oakwood cats. It was a very friendly cat. I was able to pet the cat, and it never looked fearful like most feral cats. I brought a kennel the next evening and caught the cat and brought it home.

I took it to the vet the next morning. The cat had no chip and the vet determined the cat was a Bengal breed. Based on his behavior, he felt the cat had been a pet. I received some medication for him and took him home.

Knowing I couldn’t keep this cat, I looked for “lost cat” postings but did not find any for Bengal cats. No one I knew was interested in adopting him.

Coincidentally, it came time for another warranty check on my car. This time, I started asking if anyone there would be interested in the Bengal cat. I showed pictures of the cat to the guys, who immediately replied that they needed to get the Parts Manager...

Dan, the Parts Manager, was called to the cashier area. He almost shrieked in awe when he saw the pictures of the Bengal. He had just lost his pet Bengal cat due to old age. Dan was extremely interested in adopting this stray cat.

So I brought the stray cat to the dealership the next day. Dan was thrilled when he actually saw him in person. Dan showed me videos of his last cat, and the similarities were striking. I was confident this was a good placement.

A few months passed, and it was time for another warranty check. When I arrived for my appointment, Dan was called. He came to the lobby with a huge smile on his face. He'd named the cat William, after the owner of the dealership.

William went on to star in video after video after video. When I returned to pick up my car, the staff at the cashier area all chimed in, verbalizing that they had seen all of William's starring roles. Dan was well-liked, so everyone tolerated the videos.

My need for dealership service appointments eventually stopped, as the mechanics in my family generally take care of all of our car-related needs.

But I'll always be grateful to the staff at the car dealership for laying the groundwork that got me hooked up with the right person, at the right time, to find the perfect forever home for William.

Six degrees of separation is the idea that all people are six or fewer social connections away from each other. In other words, you can connect any two people on Earth through a chain of "friend of a friend," through a network of six acquaintances...and, perhaps, cats!

Happiness often sneaks in through a door you didn't know you left open.

- John Barrymore

Skylar

Skylar is a rare light in jail nursing—steady, brilliant, and deeply compassionate. She catches what others miss, calms crises, and treats every inmate with dignity. Working beside her reminds me what true nursing is: skill guided by a fearless, generous heart.

If you had told me that one of the most competent, compassionate, and brilliant nurses I'd ever work with would be someone I met in jail, I might have laughed. But that's exactly what happened at Oakwood Medical.

Skylar didn't just stand out—she glowed.

I remember the first time I worked a shift with her. She walked into the med room like she'd been born for this. A calm confidence radiated from her, and she greeted every staff member with a warm smile and a quick, "How are you holding up today?"

"Skylar," I said that day, pulling a fresh printout of the med pass list from the printer, "I hope you're ready. Dorm C is a zoo this morning."

She glanced at the list and gave me a sideways smile. "Isn't it always? Let's go tame it."

Skylar had joined Oakwood after spending years at a prison with a high mental health population. That experience made her uniquely comfortable in the jail setting. She could walk into a pod of recently booked inmates—some still detoxing, others experiencing psychosis—and speak to them with a calm, steady voice that somehow reached them through all the noise in their heads.

One evening, we were dealing with a man who had just come in off the street, obviously deep in alcohol withdrawal. He was pacing, agitated, drenched in sweat.

"He didn't get his morning dose," a deputy told us. "He said he felt weird, then started throwing up."

"Let me talk to him," Skylar said softly.

She approached the man carefully, crouched just a bit to get to his eye level.

"Mr. Garcia?" she said gently, her voice steady. "I'm Nurse Skylar. You're going to be okay, but we need to check on your meds."

"I'm burning up," he muttered, swaying. "My skin's on fire..."

She reached out, palms open. "I know. It feels scary. We're going to help. But I need to see your chart."

Back in the med room, she started scrolling through his electronic record and frowned.

"Look at this," she said, pointing to the screen. "This taper isn't complete. He should've had a midday dose of Librium. It's missing."

She clicked through a few more windows. "No order for it at all. That's dangerous. If he misses another dose, he could suffer a seizure."

I called the on-call MD while Skylar charted the update. We caught the mistake just in time, and the medication was administered within minutes.

That kind of attention to detail in a jail setting is rare. You're constantly being pulled in 10 directions, dealing with everything from medication passes to wounds to psych evals, all with limited time and under constant security surveillance. In just one dorm, med pass can take two hours or more. But Skylar never let the chaos get to her.

Another time, during a late shift, she noticed a young man limping as he approached the pill line.

"You okay, Mr. Bennett?" she called.

"S'all right, nurse. Just a sore foot."

"Let me see," she said. "Now."

He hesitated, but she was already rolling over a stool. When he sat and pulled off his sock, we saw an angry red swelling on his heel.

"This is an abscess," she said immediately. "How long's this been like this?"

"A couple of days. They told me to go to sick call."

"Forget sick call," Skylar said. "We're treating it now."

She got on the phone with the on-call MD and secured an order for antibiotics and a warm compress regimen. Had she waited, that infection could have spread by morning.

What really set Skylar apart, though, is how she treated the inmates. Some of our coworkers—good nurses, but hardened by years in corrections—carried judgmental attitudes.

"They're here for a reason," one nurse once said with a shrug.

But Skylar didn't see it that way.

"Everyone deserves care," she'd say. "Doesn't matter where they are."

She proved that every day. One morning during med pass, she spotted an older inmate sitting alone, looking confused.

"Mr. Raymond!" she called out cheerfully. "Did you eat today?"

He shook his head. "Didn't feel like it."

"You take your meds this morning?"

"I think so. Maybe not."

She walked over and crouched beside him.

"Let me ask you something, Mr. Raymond. Do you know what your blood pressure meds are for?"

"To, uh...slow my heart?"

"Close!" she said with a warm laugh. "They help lower the pressure in your blood vessels so your heart doesn't have to work so hard. Let's make a deal—you take them after breakfast, every day. And I'll see if we can move your med time later so you don't miss it again. Sound good?"

He smiled, the first I'd seen from him in days.

She'd do this constantly—teaching diabetic patients about sugar control, reminding inmates with wounds how to care for them, quizzing guys in the pill line about their meds.

"What does Lisinopril do?" she asked one man as she handed him his dose.

"Blood pressure," he answered confidently.

"And side effects?"

"Dry cough," he grinned. "You already told me last week."

"That's right!" she said, beaming.

I'd seen Skylar shout down a hallway to a hard-of-hearing patient, just to make sure he got his meds, and I'd seen her walk out of her way to follow up with a guy who hadn't shown up for his appointment. And she did all of it without complaint—always smiling, always present.

Skylar is the kind of nurse who used her clinical training with the precision of a surgeon, but also her heart, with the gentleness of a mother, and the wisdom of someone who's seen it all. Working beside her was more than a privilege. It was an inspiration.

If the patient had trouble getting up in the morning, Skylar would ask the doctor if their medication administration time could be changed, so the patient could be more compliant with their medication. She could be heard teaching patients about elevated blood pressure, wound healing, diabetic care, and medication effects and side effects. It was quite disheartening to hear how many inmates can't name the medications they are currently taking. Many did not know why they were taking certain medications. But Skylar could be heard quizzing her patients on their medications. It was music to my ears. She was a nurse who used her training, but also her heart, to provide the highest quality of care to her patients.

In a place where so many walls go up between patients and providers, between compassion and control. Skylar reminds us what true nursing looks like: skill guided by a fearless, generous heart.

> ***Love is the most important thing in the world, but baseball is pretty good, too.***
>
> \- Yogi Berra

Six Degrees of Separation of a Borrowed Breast Pump

When Judy told me about Valerie—a young mother struggling to pump milk for her newborn while in custody—my heart cracked. She'd been borrowing pumps wherever she could, as if motherhood were a privilege she had to beg for. Judy fought through layers of bureaucracy, refusing to let herself be forgotten. Watching her advocate so fiercely for one small, life-changing piece of equipment reminded me that in jail, change often begins with one stubborn, caring soul who won't give up.

I talk to a lot of people. Most of the stories in this book began coming together that way, with a conversation. At Oakwood, I talked to coworkers, inmates, deputies, janitors, and doctors. I talked to the family members who called in to check on their loved ones. I talked to chaplains, dentists, psychiatrists, and psychologists.

Outside of work, I talk to people, too. At the gym, the grocery store, the funeral home, hair salon, among others. People have interesting things to say, if you're willing to listen.

This particular story started with a conversation with Judy from Mental Health. The MH team had always helped me understand why inmates did some of the unusual things they did. Especially the things that didn't make sense on the surface. As a nurse, my job was physical: checking blood sugar, giving insulin, changing wound dressings. But mental and emotional wounds? That was their arena.

Some Mental Health staff didn't feel safe talking to inmates directly. They'd do what we called a "drive-by": speaking through the locked door of a cell and keeping it quick.

Not Judy. She waited until the inmates were locked down, then asked the deputy to open a cell door so she could meet with someone privately in a secure room. Judy didn't judge. She listened. And the inmates knew it. When Judy interacted with someone, they walked away feeling heard. That alone is rare in jail.

"Can I Talk to You Tonight?"

About a year and a half before I retired, I was working a busy shift as Charge Nurse, juggling the usual chaos, when I saw Judy walk into Medical. She had just finished her weekly Trauma Recovery group with the women in medium security. It was one of her favorite parts of the job.

She came over and asked quietly, "Nancy, can I talk to you tonight?"

"Of course," I said. "I'll come find you on my dinner break."

I thought she wanted to decompress. Perhaps discuss something challenging from the group. I had no idea the story she was about to tell would take me on a roller coaster ride I could have never imagined.

Valerie

When I got to the Mental Health office, Judy pulled me into a quiet corner.

"I know you care about the inmates getting decent care," she began. "That's why I wanted to tell you what's been going on with Valerie."

Valerie was a woman in her twenties who was arrested while she was pregnant, then had delivered her baby six weeks ago in custody. The usual procedure when an inmate returns to jail (without her baby, of course) is that the nurse will ask if she is interested in breastfeeding.

Oakwood Medical has a program through which equipment is supplied, i.e., a breast pump and plastic bags to fill with breast milk. The breastfeeding program costs Custody Health services nothing, as all the supplies are donated. Breast milk can be pumped, bagged, and then stored in the freezer for up to 72 hours. A crucial part of the breastfeeding program is a family member/friend who must routinely come with a cooler to pick up the frozen breast milk for the baby. Many of these ladies have no one who will do this for them. The number of bags pumped and the number picked up are documented on Medical's 24-hour report.

But Valerie had the trifecta: general family support, complete with family members who agreed to care for the newborn, and were committed to coming to Oakwood every 72 hours to pick up the milk for weeks. She was doing everything right.

"It still gets to me," I told Judy. "These women go to the hospital to have a baby and come back empty-handed. I know why. I do. But it still breaks my heart every single time."

Judy nodded. "Valerie wanted to pump breast milk for her baby. She signed up for the program. The nurse on duty placed a request for a large breast pump. She needed one bigger than the standard kind."

"Okay," I said slowly. "So, what happened?"

"She never got the breast pump," Judy said. "She had to borrow one." Someone in her pod was pumping and dumping their breast milk. Valerie used the borrowed pump to produce milk, which the deputies put in the refrigerator.

"What?" I blinked. "You're kidding."

Judy said to me that Valerie had shared in the Trauma Recovery group about her efforts to get a breast pump. "She said she'd asked every nurse she saw in her dorm. Nothing. She was trying to advocate for herself, but you know how it is. A lot of these women come from abuse. They're used to not being heard."

I nodded. "So, what did you do?"

"I went to the Nurse Manager," Judy said. "Explained everything. He said she'd get the pump."

"And?"

"The next week, after the Trauma Recovery group, I asked Valerie again. Still no pump. Still borrowing one. So I went back to the Nurse Manager again. Same response. He said she'd get it."

She paused, exasperated. "Third week, same story. No pump. So I went over his head. I reported it to the Nurse Manager at the downtown jail."

The Turning Point

That did the trick. The downtown manager was furious. She immediately called the Charge Nurse at Oakwood and ordered, "This patient needs a breast pump. Today."

Two hours later, the pump arrived. But then things took an even stranger turn...

A deputy called Medical and said, "The pump's here, but the nurse won't give it to the patient."

I stared at Judy. "You're kidding."

"I wish I were," she said. "That call got passed to the supervisor. Total madness."

Ultimately, Valerie got her own large breast pump.

The Mattress Room

I was still trying to process that when Judy added, "There's one more thing." Judy's face darkened.

"Valerie told me that Kay, one of the Day Shift nurses, pulled her out of the dorm after she finally got her own breast pump. Took her to the mattress room."

"No cameras," I said.

"Right. No witnesses. Then Kay *yelled* at her. Valerie didn't even understand why, just that she was being scolded. She was scared and humiliated."

I clenched my jaw. "And what did Kay write in the chart?"

Judy sighed. "She documented that *Valerie* yelled at *her.*"

That's when I felt something inside me snap. Valerie was a trauma survivor. She'd already lived through God knows what before jail. Now here she was, trying to do something good for her child, and we—*we*—were making it harder.

"She doesn't have the strength to file a grievance," Judy said. "Not after everything. She barely got the courage to tell me."

I sat in silence.

Eventually, the issue went all the way up to the Custody Captain. But by then, the damage was done.

Reflection

This is one story. One woman. One breast pump.

But it's just not about the pump. It's about how easy it is to dismiss someone who doesn't have a voice. It's about what happens when people in power ignore the cries of someone who's just trying to do the right thing.

Valerie didn't have a baby in her arms. She didn't have money or status. She only had her determination to care for that baby, the only way she still could.

Thank God for people like Judy, who listened. Who cared. Who didn't give up.

We need more of that.

As it turned out, this story didn't stop there. It even piqued the interest of the County Executive!

> ***Write what you know. Writing is easy.***
> ***All you have to do is***
> ***cross out the wrong words.***
>
> \- Mark Twain

Reporting to the County Executive

Valerie's breast pump weighed heavily on me. I shared the story with a friend whose daughter worked for the County Executive, never expecting it to lead to a formal meeting. I prepared carefully and sat at a long table, palms damp, speaking for women who had no voice in rooms like that. I shared my account and concerns about inmate healthcare. Walking out, I felt a rare surge of purpose—like someone beyond our walls had finally heard us.

I couldn't stop thinking about Valerie. It had been two weeks, and I was still upset about how she'd been treated, waiting endlessly for her own breast pump just to get milk to her newborn. I never got assigned to her dorm, but if I had known the full story, I would've made sure she had that pump immediately.

One afternoon, I took my friend Gizelle out for her birthday lunch. After some light chatting, I suddenly blurted out, "You won't believe what happened to one of our patients at the jail."

She looked up, surprised. "What happened?"

"An inmate just had a baby. She wanted to send breast milk to her baby, and her family was willing to come pick it up! But it took weeks for her to get a breast pump. Weeks! And no one helped her—not until Mental Health stepped in." Meanwhile, she had to borrow one.

Gizelle was horrified. "You've got to be kidding me. That's outrageous!"

"I know," I sighed. "If I had known everything she was dealing with, I would've raised hell."

A week later, I was leaving my hair appointment when my phone rang. It was Gizelle, and she was practically yelling.

It took me a minute to understand that she told her daughter Ginger, who happens to be the Executive Assistant to the County Executive, responsible for the coordination of work throughout the County in all departments, both elective and appointive. I had met Ginger several times, and I really liked her.

"Gizelle? What's going on?"

"I told Ginger what happened!" she said. "And, oh my God, she wants you to talk to her boss!"

"Who's her boss?" I asked, confused.

"The County Executive!" she shouted. "The Big Boss!"

I froze. "Wait. The County Executive? You want me to talk to him?"

Suddenly, Ginger was on the phone.

"Hi," she said warmly. "Gizelle told me about your patient. I think it's something my boss needs to hear directly—from someone who was there." She continued, explaining that her boss needed to hear about the problems with inmates not receiving adequate care at the jail. He would be very interested in the details.

I was stunned. "You really think he'd want to meet with me?" I was in shock and momentarily at a loss for words. I have always been a patient advocate, and this was an unimagined dream come true!

"I know he would," she said. "We need to know what's really happening at the jail. Let's get a meeting on the books."

When I hung up after talking to Ginger, I sat in my car, completely dazed. I've always been a patient advocate, always willing to take things up the chain of command. But this—this was new territory. I had never spoken to someone with this much power before.

At Oakwood, patient care issues often got brushed aside. It wasn't like hospice, where our CEO was brilliant, kind, and deeply involved. She made staff feel heard. But at the jail? You were lucky if you got a reply to your email.

I also used to advocate for staff. If I heard someone had been put in an unsafe situation, I'd get the facts and report it to the nurses' union. A lot of staff were too scared to speak up. But I wasn't.

Still, this meeting felt monumental.

Ginger followed up a few days later.

"It'll take a few weeks to get on the calendar," she said. "But I'll be there with you."

"Oh, thank God," I said. "Yes, please."

"Just a few things," she added. "My boss has three rules for meetings like this: no over-the-top emotion, no name-calling, and just the facts."

"Got it," I said. "Just the facts." I had to prepare!

For the next few weeks, I prepared obsessively. I started drafting notes for a 30-minute talk. I practiced with my family to make sure everything was clear and I followed Ginger's rules.

I even made appointments to feel more confident. I got my hair done. At the dentist, I told them about the upcoming meeting, and they sent me home with teeth whitening trays to make sure I'd look my best.

One day at work, I saw Judy and told her what had happened.

"They finally got Valerie her own breast pump. But it was Mental Health who made it happen, not Medical. And, I've got a one-on-one meeting with the County Executive."

Judy was shocked. "That's awful! I can't believe it took that long. This is a great chance to let someone in power know what's really happening."

The morning of the meeting, I barely slept. My stomach was in knots. My husband drove me downtown because I couldn't focus on anything but my notes.

We took the elevator up to the top floor. I gave my name at the desk, and a moment later, Ginger came to get me. She walked me through a hallway to a massive office.

Inside, the County Executive was waiting.

"Nice to meet you, Nancy," he said as we sat down at a large conference table.

He seemed like a regular person, but my nerves didn't care. My mouth was dry, and my heart was pounding.

I took a breath and opened my notebook. "Thank you for seeing me. I want to tell you about a patient at the jail who waited weeks for a breast pump."

I told Valerie's story clearly, calmly. I made sure to highlight that it was the Mental Health staff who'd stepped in, not Medical. I didn't raise my voice or point fingers. Just the facts.

I had planned for 30 minutes, but I spoke quickly and finished in 15.

He listened closely. Then he asked, "May I keep your notes?"

"Of course," I said, handing them over.

I don't remember much else. It was like an out-of-body experience. Walking out of that building, I felt a rare surge of purpose. Like, for once, someone beyond our walls had heard us. Looking back, I still can't believe it happened. Speaking to the most powerful person in the county about a neglected patient in jail? That was a dream come true for a patient advocate like me.

I never found out if anything changed because of that meeting. But it didn't matter. I got to use *my voice*. I got to speak the truth in a place where it could actually make a difference. I knew this would be a story I would never forget. These are the kind of things that happen when I talk to people. And this particular experience had an epic outcome!

Just yesterday, I had lunch with Gizelle again. I had sent her a draft of this chapter.

"You know, Nancy," she said, "in the story, you mention how much you talk to people. But what I've always admired is how well you listen."

I smiled. "Well, I've been listening to patients for decades. That's a big part of being a nurse."

It's true. Listening is how stories like Valerie's are heard, and how they're finally told.

This is key to a complete nursing assessment. I guess I take my skills off the job, too.

> ***Hearing is listening to what is said.***
> ***Listening is hearing what isn't said.***
> \- Simon Sinek

Maia

Maia was joy in the chaos of jail nursing—skilled, compassionate, and endlessly energetic. Fluent in Spanish, she cared and translated with equal empathy. Patients trusted her; coworkers relied on her. She made even concrete walls feel lighter. Years after we retired, finding her again felt like a quiet truth: some connections never fade—they simply wait.

Maia came to Oakwood from my beloved Medical Center, where she had thrived on a fast-paced Telemetry unit. From the moment she arrived, you could feel the difference—her energy was electric. She didn't *walk* through Medical housing—she *skated*, a blur of scrubs and purpose. Minimum, lockdown, the ladies' dorms—she was everywhere, doing everything.

"I'm used to running all day," she told me once, laughing as she organized a medication cart while simultaneously giving directions to two patients. "If I sit down too long, I forget how to function."

She wasn't kidding.

Maia's organizational skills were nearly supernatural. She could chart, prep meds, translate, troubleshoot, and reassure patients—all at the same time. Her multitasking wasn't frantic, though. It was smooth, seamless. Like she was born for this kind of work. She made everything look easy.

And then there was her laugh. Loud, sincere, contagious.

"Maia's on shift?" someone would ask.

"Just listen," I'd reply. "You'll hear her before you see her."

She had this deep, melodic laugh that bounced off the concrete walls of Oakwood and made the place feel just a little lighter. Even on the hardest days, it reminded you that joy could still exist here.

Being fluent in Spanish made her even more indispensable. At least once an hour, someone would pop their head into the nurses' station: "Maia, can you translate?"

Without fail, she'd nod and say, "¡Claro que sí!" and head off down the hall without a trace of hesitation. She translated with empathy, cared with heart, and moved through every unit as if purpose itself propelled her.

The Spanish-speaking patients adored her. She didn't just translate words—she explained, comforted, and advocated. One patient, an older woman with diabetes and barely a word of English, once told me through tears, "Ella me entiende. No sólo las palabras, sino a mí." *She understands me. Not just the words, but me.*

And that was Maia. Whether she was teaching a patient how to manage their insulin or explaining why they couldn't skip wound care, she did it with equal parts knowledge and heart.

Her patient care skills were up to date, and she could be heard teaching patients about their medications and the importance of compliance with diabetic call, wound care, and pill call. Maia was a coworker who delivered the highest level of patient care with her knowledge and skills (even though she giggled when she heard my feeble attempts at translating for Spanish-speaking patients). I always checked to make sure the patient understood what I was saying. I know it came from her heart.

Even after a full shift, she was often the one to stay behind if the next crew was short.

"Maia, are you *sure* you're staying again?" I asked her once, seeing her throw on another pair of gloves as the evening shift stumbled in behind schedule.

She just smiled. "I've got energy left. Besides, you know how I am. Gotta keep moving!"

She was a force.

Now, I'll admit—my Spanish is...let's just say, a work in progress. I tried, though. When no one else was available, I did my best to communicate.

Once, after a particularly rough attempt to explain a medication schedule to a patient, I turned around and saw Maia leaning against the doorframe, arms crossed, trying, but *failing,* to suppress a laugh.

"Don't laugh!" I said, chuckling to myself. "I checked with him three times to make sure he understood!"

Maia wiped tears of laughter from her eyes. "You told him his pills were '*muy confundido.'* I think you meant 'muy importante.'"

We both cracked up. But there was never any judgment—just affection. She appreciated that I tried. That was Maia: she expected effort, not perfection.

After I retired, I missed her. We drifted apart, as people do when work is no longer the thread connecting them. Time passed, and I often thought about her. But life moved on.

Then, one day, the Universe stepped in.

I was visiting a friend who had recently undergone a quadruple bypass. He was recovering at a skilled nursing facility I'd never been in. It took some time to find the place, and longer still to figure out the layout. I eventually located his room and stayed a while, chatting, checking in, and gently critiquing the care without being too obvious about it.

I remember thinking, *Maybe I should've worn scrubs...just to signal that this patient has medical people watching over him.* It sounds silly, but sometimes I think the smallest things can make a difference.

After the visit, I made my way to the reception desk to sign out. I was halfway through scribbling my name when someone approached beside me.

"Hey," a familiar voice said, casual and light.

I looked up. And stared.

"Maia?" I asked, almost breathless.

She grinned. "Yes! It's me!"

"You're kidding me," I said, blinking, my brain trying to catch up. "Is it really you?"

"It's really me," she said, her smile lighting up the whole lobby. "I work here on weekends."

Of course she did. Maia never slowed down.

We stood there, grinning, hugging, catching up in a flurry of "How have you been?" and "You look exactly the same!" and "What are the odds?"

And then, as quickly as she appeared, she was off again.

"I've got a wound dressing to change," she said, slipping back into nurse mode. "But I'm *so* glad I saw you."

I walked out of that building in a haze of joy. My heart felt full. I looked up at the sky and said, out loud, "Thank you."

Because sometimes, the Universe sends you exactly what you didn't know you were missing.

And sometimes, it comes wrapped in scrubs and laughter, with a name tag that says *Maia.*

> ***The past does not repeat itself,***
> ***but it rhymes***
>
> \- Mark Twain

The Day I Felt Safer at Oakwood Than at Home

One morning, I looked out the kitchen window and froze—SWAT vehicles, deputies with rifles, reports of an active shooter. My quiet street had turned into a tactical nightmare. My hands shook as I checked on my family, my mind flipping through worst-case scenarios. For the first time, home felt more dangerous than the jail I'd once feared. The irony stung: I felt safer behind bars. It was later ruled a misunderstanding—target practice. Another false alarm followed two years later. The lesson lingered deeper each time: everyday life is wildly, quietly unpredictable.

One beautiful summer day, I was packing my lunch, getting ready to go to work (3-11:30 p.m. shift). The windows to our house were open. A comfortable cool breeze floated in through the screens, carrying with it the scent of dry grass from the foothills east of Oakwood, where we live. It was normally a 10-minute drive to work (unless a deer tried to cross the road).

I was smoothing the wrinkles from my scrubs when I heard the distant sound of sirens. "Do you hear that?" I asked my husband.

He set down his coffee. "Yeah...must be something in town. I'll check." As president of our volunteer fire department, he always had an ear tuned to emergency radio frequencies. Static filled the room. But after flipping through the channels, he shook his head. "Nothing. No calls, no dispatch." The sirens rose again, then faded. Again, and again. Eventually, we chalked it up to the wind carrying the sound from miles away.

An hour later, I left for work on time, kissed hubby goodbye, and started my drive. Just one straightaway and two curves down our narrow hill, I slammed on the brakes. Red and blue lights flashed in the shadows of oak trees. A wall of sheriff's vehicles lined both sides of the road — at least two dozen of them. Deputies in bulletproof vests, helmets, shields, and riot gear moved in clusters, automatic rifles angled against their chests, staged for action. My pulse hammered. Rifles. I'd seen helmets and shields at Oakwood during emergencies — but never automatic weapons.

I rolled down the window, heart in my throat. "What's going on?" I called to the nearest deputy. He didn't look at me. Just lifted a hand, signaling me to keep driving. A lump formed in my throat as I crept forward.

A few neighbors were pulled to the side, engines idling, windows down, waiting to drive home. I leaned toward one familiar face. "Do you know what's happening?" I asked. They said they had heard something about an "active shooter" somewhere up the hill. I was mortified!

I knew I couldn't go back home to warn my family, so I continued down the hill until I got a signal on my cell and called home. "Don't go outside," I blurted out to my husband when he answered. "Keep everyone inside. Something's happening: sheriffs everywhere, guns out."

We had lived here for nearly 30 years, and nothing like this had ever happened before.

Continuing my drive to work, I passed a massive black military-style vehicle from a nearby city headed up the hill toward the incident. White bold block letters written on the side screamed SWAT. My breath caught. I'd never seen one before. The sight of it, hulking and unstoppable, sent my stomach lurching. I said a quick little prayer, "*Please, God, keep them safe. Keep us all safe.*"

By the time I passed through Oakwood's parking lot, I was gripping the steering wheel so tightly my knuckles ached. For the first time in my life, I realized I felt safer inside prison walls than I did in my own neighborhood.

The gate deputy raised an eyebrow as I signed in. "Rough drive in?" I couldn't hold it in. "They're in my neighborhood," I blurted. "Sheriffs everywhere. Rifles. SWAT. My husband's home, and I can't get back to him. Nobody will tell me what's happening. What if—what if—"

"Hey." His voice softened. "I'll keep an ear out. They encrypt radio traffic on secure channels when it's dangerous. I'll let you know what I hear." Hours passed. Every time the phone rang in Medical, I jumped.

Finally, the deputy called. "False alarm," he said. "New neighbor called 9-1-1, and told them he thought it was a machine gun. Turned out it was just target practice. Legal out there. No one hurt."

Relief washed over me so suddenly that I had to steady myself against the counter. I thanked him again and again, but the truth was, my nerves would take days to settle.

Two years later, a similar incident happened again. This time, trucks from the volunteer fire department and city emergency services lined our road, lights flashing. Traffic stopped at our driveway. "Now what?" my husband muttered, watching from the porch. He got the call on his fire department radio — a woman screaming, along with gunshots. The words tasted all too familiar.

When the truth came out, it bordered on absurd. The "screaming woman" was a peacock! The gunshots? A retired police lieutenant was trying to scare pesky birds away from his orchard.

Still, I'll never forget the sight of my neighbors — confused, frightened, health already fragile — facing down a SWAT team with weapons drawn.

After that, neighbors began sending out reminders: *Call us first before you shoot your guns.*

Because, in our little corner of the foothills, even peacocks and target practice can summon chaos. And sometimes, Oakwood's walls felt steadier than home.

> *Flowers grow back, even after they are stepped on.*
> ***So will I.***
>
> - - author unknown

A Different Kind of Contraband

I'll admit, I slipped in small kindnesses—holiday socks, roses for Mother's Day, hummingbird trinkets, someone brought a miniature deep fryer for funnel cakes. Not all of it was legal, but all of it was human. Once, when a nurse left keys behind a locked barrier, I got approval for my husband to deliver wire cutters and wire—dangerous contraband—so a sergeant could retrieve the keys. But nothing compared to the night we smuggled in a trembling newborn kitten and found him a safe, loving home. Sometimes contraband was exactly what the heart required.

Deputies are constantly challenged by contraband. The deputies can perform "shakedowns" if there is sufficient staffing. The process begins by moving the inmates away from the area to be searched. Officers remain with the inmates while this happens.

All containers, bedding, books, and other items each inmate has in their cell are checked by more deputies for items they aren't allowed to possess. Sometimes the deputies find contraband. In the Oakwood Administration building is a collection of items found during shakedowns. A closed case with glass doors has all of the fake "Hummel" figurines made by inmates out of soap. They are "painted" with the colors of Skittles obtained from commissary. There is also a case full of "shanks."

Contraband rules (and penalties for breaking the rules) also apply to staff.

I began bringing my assortment of contraband after I worked at Oakwood for 10 years. It started with pins and bracelets for Halloween. Then progressed to sneaking in flowers for Mother's Day. Most of my ladies spent several Mother's Days in jail without any visitors. I didn't know the details of their situations, but I felt like trying to cheer them up a little when I had to work on Mother's Day.

I put the flowers in my backpack with my dinner and cat food (to feed the feral cats after my shift) and hoped the deputy at the gate where staff entered the building wouldn't check my bag too closely. I'd also found a water bottle, cut it in half, put some water in it, and added four roses from the local grocery store florist department. I added an essential oil scent to give it a "rose" scent. I placed it on my medicine cart for evening pill call. The deputies in the dorm were pretty laid back and didn't complain. When the sergeant came in, I would place medicine bottles around it. The ladies saw the roses, smelled the rose scent, and really enjoyed the flowers. My ladies in the high security dorm had not seen flowers for years. Seeing and touching a rose was a big deal. I had to watch and make sure no one took a petal of the rose.

Another type of contraband someone brought to Oakwood was a small deep fryer and oil to make funnel cakes with the nurses during the summer. My kids were in 4H when they were growing up, so our family went to the Fair every year. When I got braces as an adult, I realized I couldn't have my usual candied apple for my Fair food indulgence. That was the first time I tried funnel cakes. I was hooked. They were yummy.

The nurses and I would plan a menu and pick a weekend during the summer when the bosses were off to hold a Funnel Cake Party. Piece by piece, someone brought the mini deep fryer during the week, so it wasn't obvious it was for a party. Uncontrolled personal appliances are not allowed.

The night of the party, we made a huge mess in the kitchen, and gorged ourselves on funnel cake for dinner. We always cleaned up so the bosses never knew what mischief we had been up to. I thought fresh funnel cake at the fair was delicious, but fresh "contraband" funnel cake in jail was a whole bunch better.

My hairdresser always decorated her shop for the holidays and each change of seasons. One spring day, I noticed she had hummingbirds in the flower decorations. I asked about them, saying my cats would love to chase a hummingbird as a toy. She promptly went to her supplies of decorations and handed me 6 little hummingbirds, all different colors for my cats. She is a very generous person. My cats played with the hummingbirds a few times.

I got an idea that the Oakwood ladies would probably love to see a little hummingbird. So I brought one to work one day. I taped it to the top of the monitor on the screen of my medication cart. The ladies loved the hummingbird.

They asked, "What's its name?" "I don't know," I replied. So, we had naming contests. It was a tiny piece of contraband that the ladies really enjoyed. I was beginning to get a reputation amongst the ladies who had been there a while as a nurse with a heart for her patients. I always made sure I took home all pieces of contraband every night.

One night, our acting shift supervisor, Mary, was having a tough night when she accidentally locked the keys to all of Oakwood Medical in her office. Not only the keys, but also the nursing schedule and their contact information were locked in the office.

Mary came out to let us know what had happened, and the Charge Nurse, I, and the supervisor tried to think of ways to unlock the door, to no avail. The supervisor called to locate the sergeant on duty. Luckily, it was everyone's favorite sergeant. He arrived in Medical a few minutes later and was taken to the locked office door. The sergeant admitted he had opened many locked doors while on foot patrol, but this was a different situation. It was Friday evening. The official "locked door specialist" would have to be called in, which would incur a hefty after-hours charge...minimum $1,000.

The sergeant thought and thought. He finally came up with the idea that if we could find a wire coat hanger, he could fashion a hook under the door to unlock it. We couldn't find one anywhere in Oakwood Medical or Mental Health. He then suggested, "The last thing I can think of is some wire and wire cutters. Where are we going to get these things at this hour?"

I quietly stepped up and said, “I know a guy.” My husband had tools of all kinds, and he was not too far away.

I shared this with our favorite sergeant. He said, “Okay. I’ll let the West Gate know these items are coming through, and I am fully aware of the situation.”

I called Hubby. He gladly brought his wire cutters and a spool of wire to Oakwood. I met him at the West Gate and thanked him for coming. I then brought them back to the sergeant, who used the wire to unlock the door in a matter of minutes. I promptly took the wire cutters and spool of wire back to the West Gate for safekeeping, as agreed, until I left that night.

It was extremely exciting for me to know I'd carried authorized wire cutters into a jail, which would be extremely dangerous contraband if they made it into the wrong hands.

Officially, nothing unexpected happened that night...The greatest sergeant got the door unlocked, and we had a fun story to tell.

This last story about contraband is very different from the others...

One of our deputies lived in a home where several feral cats hung around the neighborhood. She always took care to feed them and get them to see a vet if they looked sick. One day, as she was getting ready to drive to work, she noticed a tiny kitten. Upon closer inspection, it looked like a newborn. She looked everywhere for its mother but was unsuccessful. Refusing to leave it out in the yard by itself, so she placed it in a kennel and brought it to work with her.

The deputy stopped by the Mental Health office on her way to start her shift and asked a staff member if she could keep an eye on the kitten for the evening. The MH staff readily agreed to the request. The deputy brought a bottle and formula to feed the kitten. Word got out pretty quickly that there was a tiny kitten in the Mental Health office. (It was after hours; the bosses were gone.) This kitten was cared for all night long.

The Oakwood staff created a rotation of members who could take this kitten home. Newborn kittens need care 24 hours/day. The kitten was brought to someone's home at night, and then brought back every day. The kitten was left in an office with windows while the Oakwood staff was in the unit. Inmates who passed by could see the kitten being bottle-fed. It really brightened up their day.

This little kitten was the cutest contraband I've ever seen at Oakwood.

This went on for several days, until my good friend's Mental Health caregiver asked if she could keep the kitten. Everyone agreed to let the kitten be adopted.

I had the kitten one last time before transferring it to its new home. My husband, a retired engineer, was in charge of kitten care that night, as I had to work. I gave him strict instructions and told him he had better take great care of the kitten. Not only did he follow my instructions, but he kept detailed hour-by-hour notes (in the form of "nurse's notes") on how much formula he'd had, if he had burped, and when the cat box was used. He kept the kitten in our bathroom so it was safe from our big dogs and cats.

We jokingly referred to this bathroom as the LORFICU (Leo O'Reilly Feline Intensive Care Unit). Since then, several newborn kittens and seniors nearing the Rainbow Bridge have spent time in this special place. It will always hold special memories for me.

> ***Focus on what you want, but never forget to be grateful for what you already have.***
> - Your Positive Oasis.com

The Feral Cat Program

The feral cats of Oakwood became part of my soul. Late at night, under buzzing lights and long fence shadows, I'd carry out bowls of food and feel a tail brush my leg. They were survivors—scrappy, resourceful, unexpectedly tender. Once, an Animal Control officer there to meet with an inmate who was arrested earlier that day nearly brought me to tears. The cats taught me what few humans do: even in captivity, love finds a way. Those bonds led me to build a Cat House at home—a sanctuary where the fragile ones could retire with dignity, far from concrete and steel.

Long before the Oakwood Correctional Facility was built, feral cats made their home on the grounds. With no one to spay or neuter them, their population grew. They performed a valuable role by controlling the rodent problem without the use of poison, doing their part to maintain balance in their environment.

Thirty years ago, rumors began to spread that the cats might be rounded up and euthanized. A small group of staff members, dedicated animal lovers, decided they couldn't let that happen. Together, they devised a plan to feed, spay or neuter, and all around care for the cats in a humane and sustainable way. A mental health therapist on staff presented their proposal to the County Board of Supervisors, and in 2000, it was officially approved. Since then, the cats have been a protected part of Oakwood's ecosystem.

I joined Oakwood Medical several years later. At first, I didn't notice the cats—probably because I wasn't looking for them. But the same therapist who launched the program had become a good friend of mine. One day, she asked, "Would you be interested in becoming a volunteer? I'm planning to retire, and I'm hoping someone can take over my part." As soon as she explained what the program was all about, I said, "Yes, I've never been able to turn my back on animals in need."

There were several feeding areas for the cats. I already knew about the spot by the women's buildings—I'd walked past it hundreds of times. But she introduced me to areas I'd never seen before, like the beautifully landscaped Captain's Garden near the staff dining room. There was a pond, lush greenery, and a sense of peace I hadn't expected to find in a correctional facility. I thought I'd seen the most attractive parts of Oakwood, but this little corner surprised me.

Volunteers were required to feed the cats after hours, after their shift was over. So my orientation took place at night. I was brought to the minimum housing area, to a place called the Information Center. It felt like Grand Central Station. All inmates going out from their housing to the grounds had to notify the deputies where they were going and why. Inmates passed through constantly. There were diabetics coming to Medical, trustees going to their different jobs, and inmates coming to Medical for an appointment, an X-ray, etc. An escort was required for the feeding area near the Chow Hall. Sometimes, when deputies needed to clear things out before someone could walk me over, I had to wait for an escort. It was always about our safety.

The first time I fed the cats by the Chow Hall, I felt like I had stepped into a park. There were large trees and carefully kept lawns (back when drought restrictions hadn't taken their toll). If I ignored the barracks off to the side, it felt like I could be walking barefoot through a peaceful garden. A quaint little chapel sat in the middle of it all, adding to the quiet charm. I remember one night, a longtime night-shift deputy told me about his favorite cat, Doc—though he called him Smokey—who would wait in the trees to greet the inmates lining up for breakfast. It reminded me that even in unexpected places, special moments happen.

Before long, I got into the rhythm of things and became pretty confident in my role. One night after midnight, I was at one of the feeding spots when I sensed someone dressed in a uniform was walking up the sidewalk behind me. I assumed it was a deputy. As I was chatting with one of the cats and leaving food, I heard a voice say, "I really like people who talk to animals."

I turned and realized it wasn't a deputy at all. It was an Animal Control officer. I was caught a little off guard and asked what had brought him there at that hour. He replied, "A homeless person was arrested yesterday, who had a kitten at the time of the arrest. I'm going to visit the inmate to see if he has a family member who could care for the kitten." I was impressed that Animal Control sent their staff to Oakwood at midnight to find a safe place for the kitten to stay while its owner was incarcerated. That stuck with me.

*　　　*　　　*　　　*

Speaking to him reminded me of a ridiculously crazy incident that took place when my friend Jen was unexpectedly hospitalized for a few days. I knew her medical team would take care of her. Her friends on social media sent many messages to support her well-being. She looked after feral cats near a beautiful older section of town. I volunteered to feed them. She gladly accepted.

That night, I parked by the curb around 12:30 a.m., after my shift. I put out the food and waited. Only one of the two cats came to eat. As I was deciding whether to leave, an older car slowly crept down the street with its dim headlights barely cutting through the darkness.

The driver was closely watching an apartment building. My instincts kicked in—I tried to get a good look at the driver in case I needed to report anything to the police. The car made a U-turn and drove past the apartments again. It was now 1:30 in the morning. After working in a jail, everyone starts to look suspicious at that time of night.

Right after the car disappeared, an Uber pulled up to the apartments, and a petite woman walked out. I was shocked by what I saw in this nice part of town. I wondered if the slow driver had hacked the Uber app and was planning something disastrous. Maybe I watch too much *Dateline*, or maybe working in a jail makes you see the world differently. Probably both.

* * * *

After I retired, I continued to feed the Oakwood cats. On one quiet evening, I made my usual rounds. I finished with the group near the women's building and moved on to check in with Andy and Intruder near Admin. I opened a can for Andy, but he wasn't impressed. He sniffed and walked away. He ran over to see what I had left for Intruder, but turned his nose up at that one, too. He was as finicky as ever.

I'd already seen two skunks earlier that evening, so I knew better than to leave any leftovers. I pulled some empty cans from my trash bag and began scooping the untouched food back up. As I focused on cleaning, I suddenly became aware of a deputy heading out of the Admin building, walking toward the gate behind me. I heard a friendly "Hi" and, with my back still turned, I instinctively replied, assuming he was speaking to me. Andy was sitting near the gate, so maybe the greeting was meant for him, too—who knows?

Then the deputy paused and called out, "Is that you, Nurse Nancy?" I turned and smiled, replying that it was indeed me. It was dark, and I couldn't make out who he was right away. But he had just finished a grueling 16-hour shift—4 hours overtime—and he still had the energy to greet me with kindness. Even more touching, he remembered me. That small gesture, at the end of a long day for both of us, meant more than he probably knew. Honestly, that little moment made my whole night. I was still smiling the next day.

A little while later, as I made my way out through the West Gate after feeding the kitties, I noticed a woman standing in line to check in with the deputy. She looked at me and said, "Are you still here?" I glanced at her curiously, and she smiled and added, "It's me—Corrine. I was here 10 years ago. Do you remember me?"

I did. Her face sparked a memory, and I believe I'd even seen her the year before, during another shift, when someone had called out, “Hi Nurse.” What a full-circle moment that was.

As I write this, I’m currently covering extra feeding shifts while people are on vacation. It’s more work, sure, but when moments like these happen—little reconnections, kind words, shared memories—it’s hard to complain. These experiences stay with me.

*   *   *   *

In the backyard behind my house, I helped my husband create a special 10x20-foot sanctuary, lovingly referred to as the Cat House. It’s filled with natural light from windows and skylights, and features a 10x10 "catio" so the animals can enjoy the fresh air and sunshine without wandering off. They have shelves and towers to climb on, and warm, heated beds for chilly nights. We even added a sally port—a kind of double-gate system like we had at Oakwood— to make sure no one escapes. It’s not just a shelter—it’s a place of peace, safety, and comfort.

Over time, I’ve grown especially attached to the older cats. They naturally grow weaker and fragile as they age. I couldn’t stand the thought of them dying alone under a bush, scared and cold. So, when the time feels right, we gently trap one and bring it home. I feed them twice a day and keep their litter boxes clean. Most importantly, they get to spend their final days in comfort, surrounded by gentle care and affection every single day. It’s a true sanctuary for their final chapter—a way to honor their lives with dignity and love. And in return, they bring a quiet, soulful presence that fills our home and hearts.

My role as a volunteer caretaker has become more than just routine—it’s a deep, heartfelt commitment. These cats have found a special place in my life, and I’ve found joy and purpose to make sure they’re safe, cared for, and loved.

> ***What greater gift than the love of a cat?***
> \- Charles Dickens

Parking Lot Adventures

Late shifts meant crossing the parking lot with newly released inmates. One woman sang to the night, certain she was the next Mariah Carey. An elderly man wandered in frightened circles until a deputy called him a taxi. Even a stray rooster found a deputy to take him home. But the night someone approached me in the dark, my pulse roaring, changed everything. I never walked out alone again.

I worked 3-11:30 pm for most of my career at Oakwood. Nurses, mental health staff, and clerks would finish our tasks (on a good night) around 11:15 pm then put things away in anticipation of leaving at 11:30 pm. One significant problem with leaving work from a correctional facility vs. a hospital at midnight is that inmates are also being released at that time. We all pass through the same door, the West Gate. The deputy in charge will usually give us a heads-up if a group of inmates has been recently released. They could be waiting in the parking lot to be picked up by a family member, or just hanging out. One time, an inmate released at night promptly broke into one of the employees' cars. He was quickly rearrested.

One evening after midnight, I walked out to the parking lot with (another) Nancy, who worked for the Department of Corrections (DOC). She issued inmates clothes to change into when they arrived at Oakwood, and returned their belongings to them when they were released.

We were both part of the small group of volunteer staff who took care of the feral cats who lived at Oakwood. We had already fed the cats. Now we were headed out to get a trap to try to catch two older cats who were getting quite thin and needed extra care.

A young woman in her 20s approached us. She had her purse and held some keys in her hand. She stopped and said, "Can you help me?" We turned to her and answered, "Yes," thinking she may need directions. She said, “My name is Melissa. I need to find my car. I can't find my car." We asked her if she had just been released. She replied, "Yes, and I can't find my car."

We told her, "But if you got arrested, your car wouldn't be here. Do you have family to call? Where are you going?"

Melissa replied, "I'm married. My husband and I live in Monte Sereno. I'm the next Mariah Carey." She sang to us in the parking lot to show off her melodious voice.

At that point, we realized Melissa probably had some Mental Health (MH) issues. She didn't seem to understand what we were talking about. And we were worried about her safety. We gently suggested that we all return to the West Gate, where all staff and inmates leave. We assured her we could get some help from the Oakwood deputy who supervised the entrance.

We entered through the door together. Melissa walked along with us, rambling about being the next Mariah Carey and finding her husband. We approached Deputy Small, a seasoned deputy. We explained, "Deputy Small, we met Melissa in the parking lot. She told us she lives in Monte Sereno. She is looking for her car in this parking lot. She is the next Mariah Carey. Can you help get her home safely?" We were hoping our description of Melissa would imply that she had MH issues and needed support.

Deputy Small replied, "Miss Melissa, I told you to go catch the bus! Now *GO GET ON THE BUS*!" Melissa quietly replied, "Okay."

Nancy and I stared at each other in total disbelief! This deputy was not willing to help this poor woman by calling his Sergeant to request a courtesy drop-off at the hospital, with which we had a contract to care for inmates. We had had sergeants okay a drop-off for other at-risk inmates at the hospital who weren't safe on their own when they were released. Melissa was probably a “new” booking, arrested the day before. MH could have arranged a taxi if they had met with her and determined she wasn't safe on her own. But we didn't question his decision. He could have made a lot of trouble for Nancy and me. We looked on with sadness as Melissa walked out the door. And we prayed that she would safely arrive at her home that night.

The next parking lot story has a better ending. A year later, working in Oakwood Medical, I saw Helen, one of the best MH staff. I was Charge Nurse and met her in Medical at the front desk. She let me know she was expecting a 74-year-old gentleman who had been referred to her following his appearance in court for displaying confusion. The older man couldn't remember that he had been to court earlier that same day. Helen was concerned for his safety in his current housing: a barracks with 60 men of all ages, with minimal supervision.

She began to put out notifications to rehouse him to another facility, where he could be more closely supervised. Then Helen found out the inmate was being released. So she re-interviewed him to determine if someone could come pick him up and give him a ride home upon his release. He assured her he would call his girlfriend for a ride. The inmate left to be processed for release.

Later that same night, I walked out at the same time as Helen. We were both leaving long after all the other staff left, so we were alone in the parking lot after midnight. We noticed an older man wandering around the parking lot. Helen recognized him as the same man she had spoken to earlier, who had assured her that his girlfriend would come pick him up.

We went to him. Helen asked him if he had called his girlfriend. He replied, “I don’t have her number after all. Things are missing from my wallet.” Indeed, his cell phone was at his residence, 20 miles away. The man asked if someone could point him to a motel, so he could make other arrangements in the morning.

Helen and I brought him back to West Gate, where Deputy Richards was working the area. Helen explained that the man was confused and had no ride home. The deputy looked in the man's wallet and found a credit card. He called for a taxi. Deputy Richards pulled up the address on his court papers and confirmed it with the man. He also copied down the cell phone number. The deputy helped the man get safely in the taxi and gave the driver the correct address. Deputy Richards called the cell two hours later and the man answered. He had made it home safely. The man's only concern was locating his girlfriend. Deputy Richards said he couldn't help him there.

Because of the few extra minutes it took Deputy Richards to arrange for a ride and follow up with a call, this man made it home safely. Helen and I both sent letters of commendation to his superiors.

One summer evening, a rooster appeared at the south end of the employee parking lot! It appeared to be missing tail feathers, but was getting around okay. It pushed the two feral cats in the parking lot out of the way to eat some of their kibble. Once word got out about a rooster in the parking lot, several employees brought food for the rooster. With its own food, it stayed away from the cats.

Attempts were made to find a rescue to come pick it up. It slept on the hood of the service vehicles parked at the south end of the lot! At 3 am, it began crowing, hence us determining it was a rooster. Inmates in the minimum camp barracks heard it. It crowed until night shift left at 6 am! But much to the surprise of the Oakwood staff, none of the inmates complained about the crowing! This was an unexpected surprise in the middle of a bustling metropolitan area. Maybe it was a reminder of simpler times. The rooster eventually found a forever home with one of the deputies.

I volunteered to feed the feral cats at Oakwood one particular night after I retired. By then, I had been feeding them for nine years while I was working, and for three years since I'd retired. When working, I would feed the cats living on the grounds inside the jail first. When I left the facility, I would drive to the end of the parking lot and feed the two cats that lived outside the security fence. Now that I am retired, when I arrive to feed the cats around 10 pm, I start in the parking lot.

This happened to be a busy weeknight; there were plenty of cars in the parking lot because there were not only staff vehicles, there were visitor's vehicles. I drove down to the end of the parking lot, put my car in Park, grabbed food and water, and left my car running with the door open because it only takes three minutes to feed, water, and say, "Hi," to the cats. Then I was back in my car to park and go feed the cats living inside the Oakwood facility. This was what I had done for the three years since I retired.

This particular night, I drove to the area where I fed the "parking lot" cats. No cameras, no staff patrolling the parking lot. I pulled around, stopped, placed my car in Park, left the car running (it is a hybrid, so sometimes it sounds off when it's on), and got out to feed the cats who were waiting for me.

While I was finishing up, a tall young man walked up to me and asked, "How do I get out of here? I need to catch the bus." I was shocked; this guy was just released from Oakwood and I'd missed seeing him walking around the parking lot! I was completely caught off guard.

I explained that there was a fence around the facility, and he would need to walk back the way he came to find the exit. Standing next to my car, he asked, "Whose car is this? Can you give me a ride?" I quickly said, "It's my car. I'm going to work after I feed the cats." He bought my story and turned around and left. I was still shaking when I got back in the car. I slowly drove to park so I could go inside and feed all the other cats. I walked into the West Gate, and he was sitting in the visitors' waiting area!

I quietly told the deputy what had happened in the parking lot; he said he would keep an eye on him. Next I got my visitor's badge and went in to feed the cats. I came back 15 minutes later, and he was gone. He'd taken off after I went in to feed the cats. The deputy asked if I would like an escort to my car. I declined the offer. I scanned the parking lot as I walked outside.

After all the "Safety Classes" I had sat through every two years at Oakwood, now I found myself in a potentially unsafe situation, with no one around, and out of the range of the cameras. Nowadays, when I pull up in the parking lot to feed the cats (scanning the area as I drive), I park my car at the end of the parking lot, turn off the engine, grab the food and water, get out, and lock my vehicle!

Every Time.

> ***Life is 10% what happens to you***
> ***and 90% how you react to it.***
> \- Charles R. Swindoll

The Night Maia Saved Me from a Locked Cell

One moment, I was grabbing supplies; the next, a cell door slammed shut—no handle, no radio, no way out. I was alone in a locked cinderblock box. When Maia realized I was missing and freed me, relief washed over me. In jail, doors close fast; sometimes, survival depends on a teammate who notices.

The Oakwood Medical/Mental Health building was originally designed with 1st-floor conference rooms, classrooms, a pharmacy, and a Medical Records room so that staff had meeting places, medications, records, a treatment room, and office supplies at hand for everyday use. The 2nd floor design included DOC offices on one side and an infirmary on the other, along with several individual cells and a couple of larger cells to house four inmates.

Over the years, the actual use differed from the design. The Infirmary at the downtown main jail was large enough to handle all County inmate infirmary patients, making the Oakwood infirmary unnecessary. So instead, the 2nd floor cells were used for medical supply storage.

Nurses treated wounds, assessed inmates involved in altercations, administered intramuscular meds, and cared for diabetic patients in the downstairs treatment room. It was located next to the deputy's station and had supplies for everything from abrasion to full cardiac arrest. Staff were assigned to restock each treatment room in all units at the facility each shift.

During this particular evening shift, I provided treatment for minimum security patients, which included scheduled medical treatment, along with "walk-ins" who'd injured themselves at work or during an altercation. Forty to sixty patients needed some form of medical care on an average night. My coworker and I had two and a half hours until we had to go to the pharmacy to begin the evening "pill call." We provided patient care and noted vital signs, sizes, and appearances of wounds, and documented other pertinent information for each on their invitations. (Invitations are sent to the inmate to inform them of the need to come to Medical for a specific reason.)

The routine went as follows: We check to ensure supplies are stocked in the treatment room for the next shift. We prep for pill call by getting over-the-counter meds lined up, pulling any opiates from the locked cabinet, and checking to make sure all the meds are pre-packed and ready to give as scheduled at bedtime. After pill call, we document patients who didn't show up for essential medications and send invitations to them to remind them to take their meds as ordered. We are on our feet for the last four hours of our shift.

I was surprised to look at the clock and find I had a few minutes free before I had to begin pill call. I thought of the new patient I had seen that night, who required a special burn dressing for his injury. It was different than the 4x4s, antibiotic ointment, and tape normally applied to injuries.

I decided to run upstairs to the storage room to get a box of burn dressing to use in the treatment room. No one is on the second floor after 5 pm...

"I'm going up to the storage room for dressings. I'll be back in time for pill call," I informed the Charge Nurse. Then I got the giant key to the storage room cell to access the medical supplies.

My normal routine was to bring a cart so I could collect more supplies and save my coworkers a trip. I would open the door and place the cart in the doorway to keep the door propped open. But I didn't bring the cart this particular night because I was just going for one box of burn dressings.

I opened the door, went in, and it closed behind me. I was trapped.

I had the key, but since it was a cell, there weren't any key holes inside (for obvious reasons). I did not have my cell phone. I was mildly anxious, but remembered that I had notified my Charge Nurse that I was going to the upstairs storage room. As time ticked by, though, my heart pounded as I realized I was utterly alone. No radio or phone, the door sealed. Minutes stretched like hours.

I looked around for the burn dressing. It took me a few minutes to find it. I glanced around at all of the supplies, thinking I might be able to fashion a tool to jimmy the lock. My anxiety won out over my creativity as I looked at dressings, normal saline bottles, syringes, urinary catheters, and tongue blades. So I sat on some boxes and waited for someone to come rescue me. As I did so, I felt my "fight or flight" response growing. There was a window in the room, so I began flashing the lights to attract attention in case someone was walking by. No luck. No one was outside at the time. I sat back down on the boxes and just waited.

After what seemed like a long time, I heard a knock at the door. It was Maia! I slid the key under the door, and she opened it.

"I asked the Charge Nurse where you were, and she said she didn't know! I knew you were probably up here getting stuff to restock supplies," Maia declared. She had returned early from her assignment and was asked to perform pill call for me because no one knew where I was. She knew better. That was when she came up to the storage room to find me.

I hugged her like I had been stranded on an island for decades. "I told her I was coming up here! What the hell!" I exclaimed. Relief flooded through me so intensely that I wanted to cry.

Maia is an amazing person and a quintessential teammate who pitches in when needed without being asked. For a long time after that, every time I saw her, I reminded her how grateful I was for rescuing me from that locked jail cell. For me, every one of the minutes was an eternity.

> ***Every accomplishment starts with the decision to try***
> - iHearts143Quotes.com

Dana's Raincoat

Dana, a spirited nurse, hurried through the halls in a clear raincoat trimmed in bright pink—whimsical, unmistakably her. A deputy once worried it made her look vulnerable, then learned it was simply what she could afford. Quietly, he bought her a sturdier coat. When I later learned he had died of cancer, I held that memory close. Kindness is a legacy, too.

My career at Oakwood wouldn't be complete without a story about one of my favorite coworkers. Dana was a force of nature—50-something, barely five feet tall, with a perpetual twinkle in her eye and energy that shifted between the intensity of a tropical storm and the calm of a quiet meadow. From the moment she joined our team as a nurse, we knew we had struck gold.

Dana was a fiercely independent single mom who faced life's struggles head-on and emerged stronger every time. She was the kind of woman who didn't wait for someone else to solve her problems. When her refrigerator broke and money was tight, she didn't panic. First, she scoured YouTube for DIY repair videos. When that didn't work, she bought an oversized ice chest and kept it stocked with ice—much to her daughter's dismay. With extra shifts at Oakwood, she saved up, and within weeks, a brand-new refrigerator stood proudly in her kitchen. The plumbing fiasco at her house was even worse—digging up the lawn, replacing pipes—but Dana handled it with the same steady grace she brought to everything.

Before Oakwood, Dana worked at a jail in the next county. She often shared stories—some harrowing, some hilarious—about the chaos of the Booking area, where overdoses were tragically common. The protocols there were different from ours, and listening to her talk about how nurses functioned in a different jail setting was always fascinating. At Oakwood, we operated under Standardized Procedures

(SPs) that dictated how we treated patients when the doctors weren't around. We could administer medications like Tylenol or Robitussin as long as the symptoms fit the SP guidelines. Anything outside those strict parameters meant an automatic trip to the ER. We had SPs for everything—UTIs, chest pain, diabetic emergencies, head injuries—and as nurses, we had to memorize them like our lives depended on them. Sometimes, it felt like they did.

After Dana had been at Oakwood for a while, she started recognizing faces—former inmates from her previous job, childhood acquaintances who had taken unfortunate turns in life. It seemed like she knew half the people who passed through our doors. And yet, she treated each one with the same level of care and professionalism, never letting personal history cloud her judgment.

Dana didn't have fancy jewelry or expensive scrubs and was very happy with that. One rainy season, Dana came to work in a clear plastic raincoat with pink trim that reached mid-thigh, complete with matching booties. She didn't have a lot of money to blow and it was obvious that she was so proud of her new acquisition. Dana looked so happy in her raincoat that I exclaimed, "That is a darling raincoat!"

That night, Officer Booker—one of our finest deputies—was working in Medical. A retired military man, Booker was a by-the-book officer, always serious about his job, always immaculate with his polished boots and ever-present dark glasses, even at night. But beneath that stern exterior was a heart of gold. Mid-shift, he pulled me aside.

He hesitated "I was thinking about talking to Dana, maybe to suggest something...different.

"That raincoat," he said, his voice low with concern. "It's just not right."

I braced myself. Booker wasn't the kind to comment on fashion, so this had to be serious. "What do you mean?" I asked.

Then, frowning, I added, "Dana doesn't have money to waste on fashion statements. She loves that raincoat."

His expression softened instantly. “Oh,” he said, clearly reconsidering. “I didn’t know. I won’t say anything.” And with that, we returned to work.

A few weeks later, I was assigned as Medical Charge Nurse. Officer Booker called me over to his desk. “I’ve been thinking about Dana and that raincoat,” he said. “I want to help her out. What’s her size?”

I was stunned. This no-nonsense, tough-as-nails deputy wanted to buy her a sturdy new coat. He didn’t just think about it—he acted on it. A few days later, he presented Dana with a beautiful blue raincoat, a gift from a man who spent his career ensuring order but never forgot the importance of kindness.

Booker retired not long after that. A couple of years later, he lost his battle with cancer. But I will never forget him—his integrity, his quiet generosity, and his unwavering commitment to those around him. People like Officer Booker were why I felt compelled to write this book. Oakwood may have been a workplace behind bars, but it was filled with people—dedicated, compassionate, hard-working people—who made even the toughest days worthwhile.

> ***There are two ways of spreading light:***
> ***Be the candle or the mirror that reflects it***
> \- Edith Wharton

Let Me In

A tense, darkly humorous moment unfolds when nurse Alex discovers a man calmly cutting into the jail with bolt cutters—only to learn the man is desperate to return after release, seeking safety and care over the chaos on the outside. This story blends disbelief, irony, and quiet sadness, ending with weary laughter that masks a deeper truth about vulnerability, institutional refuge, and the strange normalcy of life at Oakwood.

Nurses at Oakwood rarely have a moment to catch their breath. Shifts are packed, and the pace is relentless. But there's always that one golden hour, a one-hour break for a meal. Some bring food from home, others make a quick run to a nearby restaurant. That's what Nurse Alex did that evening.

He had just picked up a sandwich and a drink from the burger place down the road and was heading back to the facility's West Gate entrance. As he neared the front fence line, something caught his eye: movement near one of the older lockdown buildings. This was before the installation of motion sensors on Oakwood's exterior fencing.

Squinting through the dimming light, he spotted a man crouched near the base of the fence, working frantically with a shiny tool in his hands.

"What the...?" Alex slowed his car and stared. "Is that guy...cutting the fence?"

Sure enough, the man was using a bolt cutter, slicing through the chain-link like he had all the time in the world. He wasn't even trying to hide!

Alex walked into the West Gate, still stunned.

"Hey!" he called out to the deputy. "There's a guy cutting through the fence out front. Near the lockdown unit."

The deputy looked up from his monitor, grinning. "What, trying to break out?"

"No," Alex said, shaking his head. "Trying to break in. I'm serious. He's got bolt cutters, and he's almost through."

The deputy laughed. "Come on, man. Who tries to get into jail?"

"I'm not kidding," Alex said, voice rising. "He's out there, plain as day, just going at it. You better check it out."

The deputy blinked, the humor draining from his face. He grabbed his radio. "Dispatch, this is West Gate. We've got a possible intruder cutting the fence on the west side near Lockdown A. Requesting immediate response."

Within two minutes, sirens blared. Lights flashed. Deputies swarmed the area, guns drawn. The man didn't resist. He dropped the bolt cutter, raised his hands, and got down on the ground without a word.

They cuffed him and led him away, confused and mumbling something about "missing his room." He was handcuffed and taken downtown to be booked.

Later, word got around.

The man had just been released from the Acute Psych unit the day before. Apparently, he'd checked himself into a motel, ordered an Uber, and asked the driver to stop at Home Depot. He bought bolt cutters. Then he had her drop him off right outside Oakwood.

The Uber driver, visibly shaken, gave her statement to the deputies. "He seemed weird, yeah, but I thought he was just nervous or something. I had no idea he was gonna cut through a prison fence!"

Back in the break room, Alex shook his head as he relayed the story to the night shift.

"So he literally went from psych ward to Home Depot, back to jail?"

"Yup," said another nurse. "Talk about a round trip."

"He could've just knocked on the door," joked a tech. "We've got open beds."

Someone else laughed. "Can you blame him? We've got movie nights, popcorn, soda... medical, dental, psych care. Way better than the streets."

The room fell quiet for a moment.

"Still," Alex said, "cutting through a fence with bolt cutters just to get back inside? That's a first."

One of the older nurses smirked. "Welcome to Oakwood."

> ***Some days, the best thing about my job is that the chair spins.***
>
> \- Anonymous

Chaplain's Women's Summit

I was terrified walking into a room of sixty incarcerated women, every stare intense and unreadable. But once I began teaching about breast exams and hygiene, I found steady ground in my nursing role. Slowly, the room changed—laughter surfaced, shoulders relaxed, women danced in Zumba and lost themselves in painting. For a moment, the jail faded. When one woman whispered, "You took me out of this place for a minute," I realized the transformation wasn't about escaping the walls, but about reclaiming humanity within them. It became one of the most meaningful experiences of my Oakwood career.

The Oakwood women's section has a small team of female chaplains available for spiritual support. The inmates gushed about the team lead, Chaplain Lorraine, like they would a saint. I was anxious to meet this remarkable woman.

When I finally got a chance to introduce myself to her, I saw the light in her eyes and felt the love in her heart that they had described. She really did seem saint-like. This devoted woman was totally dedicated to helping these ladies in any way legally possible.

Chaplain Lorraine was usually running in the opposite direction whenever I saw her, but one day she approached me with an invitation.

She was planning a Women's Summit: a two-day weekend for the medium security ladies who don't have access to many programs. The summit would consist of several different types of classes addressing health, stress reduction, safety, exercise, and job skills. She asked if I would be interested in speaking to them about health. I jumped at the chance to be part of this life-changing experience. She asked if I knew any Zumba instructors who might be interested to come teach the ladies about dancing. I knew several instructors whom I could recommend to be part of the weekend.

On the first day of the summit, I was assigned to give my talk on health in one dorm while other volunteers were assigned to the two other dorms with different topics. So I was inside the dorm, walking around teaching basic health concepts: breast self-exams, oral hygiene, and STDs. I was used to speaking with patients one-to-one at pill call or during assessments. I knew most of them from pill call, diabetic call, wound care, blood pressure checks, or neuro checks after fights. It was somewhat disconcerting to speak to 60 inmates all at once inside the dorm. This activated "fight or flight" reactions in me. In this state, physiological changes are activated to give the body increased strength and speed in anticipation of fighting or running. Some of these changes include increased blood flow to muscles to make quick action easier, increased blood pressure and heart rate to enhance cardiac output to supply the body with more energy, increased blood sugar (glucose) secreted by the liver to provide the body with extra fuel, and increased respiration to supply the oxygen necessary to help burn the extra glucose. In addition to extra speed and strength, the pupils dilate to let in more light, allowing for better vision of the body's surroundings for a quick "fight or flight."

The whole time I spoke, the deputies made themselves visible to remind the inmates to follow the rules and stay on their bunks. So I calmed down and ran through my notes, with a few minutes to spare. I was in my element as a nurse. Teaching patients about maintaining good health is what I do. And those women were a captive audience. I asked if there were any questions, and there were a few. Some questions I could answer, and some I could not. I took names so I could follow up and get back to them with answers. It was important to me to give feedback, even if I couldn't find an answer.

There was one session where I didn't have to speak, so I joined my Zumba instructor for a fun class. She kept it basic and safe because these inmates don't get a lot of exercise. Entering the crowded dorm triggered my usual "fight or flight" response, but the music and dancing quelled my fears. I'm used to running into a dorm to attend to a medical emergency, and for one patient at a time.

The ladies in all three dorms loved the Zumba classes. It was a brilliant idea; Chaplain Lorraine had to include exercise for them. A few of them would remind me years later that they still remember how much fun they had in the Zumba class.

The second day of the summit continued like the first day. Inmates learned about safe decision-making, drawing with pens as a form of stress reduction (with supervision because pens were forbidden as potential weapons or tattoo-etching tools), and exercising to Zumba. Watching them come to life during this weekend was inspiring. For two days, I witnessed transformation – not because the walls opened, but because we did. Watching these women laugh, learn, and feel human again was meaningful. Chaplain Lorraine really loved these women. And this weekend helped give them a glimmer of hope in an otherwise challenging situation.

A group of ladies created a mural that read, "Listen, Hope, Laugh, Life." One said, "You took me out of this place for a minute. For a moment, I was free."

The Chaplain's Women's Summit provided education, faith, and support system opportunities so the ladies could plug into them when they were released. This program was one of the most rewarding opportunities I experienced in my years at Oakwood Medical.

> ***Try to be a rainbow in someone's cloud.***
>
> \- Maya Angelou

Named in a Lawsuit

The day the lawsuit papers arrived, my hands shook so badly I had to sit down. I had followed every protocol, yet my name appeared beside "negligence" and "malpractice" after a patient lost his foot. For years, the case followed me into my dreams, and into my sense of self. Even after I was cleared, the fear lingered, quietly reshaping how I saw myself as a nurse.

It started like any other day. An older man in his sixties, diagnosed with Type 1 Diabetes Mellitus, self-surrendered and was booked into Oakwood custody. Self-surrender usually happens after an individual has been through the court process and received their sentence. The court allows them time to get their affairs in order. As nurses, we're trained to handle these admissions. His paperwork was in order, with medical history and meds documented. He was housed in minimum security. His medications were promptly started—nothing out of the ordinary.

Two days later, he hobbled up to the nurse's station.

"Something's wrong with my foot," he said, his voice low but laced with worry.

That set off a chain reaction. Foot wounds and complications can spiral fast, especially for an insulin-dependent diabetic. I ordered wound care immediately and got an urgent MD appointment scheduled. We did twice-daily assessments, per standardized procedures. Still, despite our best efforts—with consultations with the Wound Specialist and the doctor appointment—his condition worsened. He was sent to the ER.

The protocols we followed were stringent, born from hard lessons learned, including a diabetic toe amputation case a decade earlier. We even had a poster in the Oakwood Medical treatment room showing the stages of wound development of a diabetic foot ulcer. I'd seen diabetic inmates stare at it, getting a reminder of what was at stake, which motivated many to keep their blood sugars stable.

Eventually, word filtered back: the patient had required multiple surgeries, and then an amputation. In the back of my mind, I thought, "Uh-oh...This isn't good."

The patient was released from custody during the hospitalization, so he never returned to Oakwood Medical.

A year passed. Then one day, I opened my mailbox to find a thick envelope from County Counsel. My heart sank. Just seeing the return address was disconcerting. Inside: a lawsuit. My name. The inmate's name. A flood of dread. Others from our team—the Wound Specialist, the doctor—were listed, too. I'd provided care there for 13 years, and now I was being sued.

Fear took hold.

"He knows where we work," I muttered to a coworker.

"Do you think he has our addresses?" None of us knew. We didn't ask.

Even when the attorney representing the custody staff told us he didn't stand a chance, the fear lingered. Every night after my 3-11 shift, everyone else working the shift left before me. I'd feed the feral cats at midnight. Alone. In the dark. No cameras. The parking lot was deserted.

I'd glance around, heart pounding, looking around the parking lot a little more than usual for suspicious behavior before diving into my car. The nurses were used to inmate releases going through the same door we used at night when we left. The deputies would give us a "heads up" if a group of recently released inmates was waiting outside. As I drove home, I watched the rearview mirror more than the road to see if I was being followed.

The other nurses named in the suit shared the same anxiety. We'd glance at strange cars, jump at unfamiliar footsteps. I watched outside my house, worried that if I ever saw a car driving by slowly, it might be the inmate who was suing us.

Our names—first and last—had been printed in the local newspaper. The lawsuit was a matter of public record. Copies of that paper were freely distributed to the inmates. One long-term inmate casually told a coworker, "I saw your name in the paper. I know who you are now."

The ancillary staff who work at Oakwood receive “hazard pay” – this is supposed to help us feel better about working in the jail setting. But even with hazard pay, it felt like there was no safety net.

One nurse was approached by an inmate who read the article and made a sarcastic comment. The nurse reported it to the sergeant, who relayed it to his Supervisor. Assignments were rearranged for nurses if inmates made comments to them about the lawsuit.

The case dragged on. The lawsuit took several years to make its way through the courts.

When the case was settled, the inmate was awarded a monetary judgment. The attorney representing us turned out to be wrong.

But that wasn’t the end of our worries. When the plaintiff is awarded a large award over a certain amount, all of the parties named in the lawsuit are investigated for malpractice.

A nurse investigator called me: "I need an updated resume. I’ll be reviewing your file and speaking with your supervisor."

I had no disciplinary actions in my record, but that didn’t ease the gnawing fear. The investigation process took over two years. It felt like ten.

I made it through. Thankfully, this was the only lawsuit I ever faced in all my years at Oakwood. Still, it left its mark. Not on my record—but on my peace of mind. Fear has a way of weaving itself into your sense of self-worth.

> ***In our lives, there are times that call for slow, gentle change, and then there are the times when you just have to let that shit go.***
>
> \- Anonymous

The Sergeant with a Heart

Sgt. Williams was steady and calm, listening without dismissal. When I voiced concern about a diabetic woman in isolation, she acted at once, ensuring every deputy understood the risk. Her quiet, unwavering support showed me how deeply custody leadership can shape patient outcomes.

Working as a nurse in a correctional facility means that no two days are ever the same. Unlike in a hospital or clinic, every shift in jail brings unexpected challenges, often unfolding in unpredictable ways. Over time, I learned that good communication with the deputies could mean the difference between routine care and a potential medical emergency.

For instance, a Type 1 diabetic who receives insulin has a medical bracelet indicating they are diabetic. The deputies need to be notified when these inmates need to keep extra food nearby in case their blood sugar drops unexpectedly. This could turn into a life-threatening situation. The deputies are taught why this is crucial for these inmates. But sometimes the issues are more complicated and need to go up the custody ladder. That is when I first met Sgt. Williams.

Sergeants have a lot of responsibility working in a jail setting. Sgt. Williams not only listened to the nurses, but she listened with her heart. She was an intelligent, caring, patient individual with a dedicated spirit for doing the right thing. No matter how crazy the shift became, Sgt. Williams took the time to listen to nurses' concerns and act upon them.

One afternoon, while reviewing the medication list, I noticed a new intake in the women's Special Management Unit – a young woman diagnosed with Type 1 diabetes. She was housed in a single cell due to her mental health history, which was not uncommon. But as I looked through her chart, something about her stood out...

"She has a medical bracelet," I said out loud, mostly to myself, "but if her blood sugar crashes, she could go unconscious within minutes."

Later that afternoon, I stopped by her cell for an initial assessment. "Hi," I said gently, peering through the glass, clipboard in hand. "I'm Nancy, the nurse on the unit today."

She sat up slowly from her bunk and came to the door. "Hi," she replied, cautiously. "Do you have any juice?"

"I can get you some if you're feeling low," I said. "But tell me more about your diabetes. Anything I need to know?"

She hesitated for a moment, then said, "I have a service dog at home. He can tell when my blood sugar's dropping...before I even feel it. He used to bark and push his nose into my leg when I was crashing. Here, it's just me."

I nodded, documenting her history with the service dog. "That's important. I'll make sure you have snacks available. But since you're alone in this cell, I want the deputies to check on you a little more often — just in case."

That's when I realized I needed backup — someone who understood the risk and could authorize enhanced checks.

I made my way to the control room, where Sgt. Williams was reviewing camera footage.

"Sargent Williams," I said, tapping lightly on the open door.

She turned, gave me a warm smile, and gestured for me to come in. "What's going on, Nurse?"

"I need your help," I said. "There's a patient in Special Management; a young woman, Type 1 diabetic. She's in a single cell and doesn't have anyone watching out for her like she would on the outside. She used to rely on a service dog to alert her to blood sugar crashes."

Sgt. Williams leaned forward, her smile fading into a serious, attentive look. "That's dangerous," she said. "How often do those crashes happen?"

"They can be unpredictable," I said. "She might look okay one minute and be unconscious the next. I suggest additional welfare checks. Maybe every 15 minutes instead of the standard 30."

Without hesitation, she nodded. "Absolutely. I'll talk to the deputies right now."

As she stood up, I added, "Thank you. I just worry about her when I'm not here."

Sgt. Williams looked at me and said, "That's why we're a team. You do your part, I'll do mine. Let's make sure she gets through this safely."

True to her word, Sgt. Williams immediately met with the deputies on duty. Within an hour, the revised check schedule was in place, and I slept better that night knowing someone was watching out for her.

Thankfully, the patient went to court a few days later and was released. No incidents, no medical emergencies. But I thought about her for days after, especially on my days off.

There were many moments over the years when Sgt. Williams stepped in, when things got tense, confusing, or downright chaotic. But that particular moment, when she didn't hesitate to adjust protocol to protect a vulnerable young woman, stayed with me the most.

I'll never forget her words: "Let's make sure she gets through this safely."

Thank you, Sgt. Williams, for your leadership, compassion, and unwavering dedication to the people of Oakwood – staff and inmates alike.

> ***The attitude you bring to the day is what the day will bring to you. Great attitude. Great day.***
> - SJ Mercury Horoscope by Eugenia Last

A Toxic Coworker

Brent altered insulin without orders, falsified documentation, and bristled when challenged. When leadership did little, I filed a Patient Safety report despite the risk of retaliation. His departure brought relief—but underscored a stark truth: incarcerated patients have no choice of their caregivers. We owe them better.

Working as a nurse at Oakwood Medical is not like working in a traditional hospital. We operate independently, in separate buildings or dorms. There's no medical supervisor down the hall to consult with, no fellow nurse to casually lean on during a rough shift. You learn to trust your training, trust the policies, and—ideally—trust your coworkers. The reality is that the last part can be the most unpredictable.

It is not unusual to work with a new nurse with no experience in correctional healthcare. They attend orientation, but the unique challenges of this environment don't always come through in those few early days. There was a time when it started to feel like the only hiring criteria were a nursing license and a pulse. That might sound harsh, but anyone who's worked in a place like Oakwood knows what I mean. When you're responsible for inmate care, you need more than competence—you also need calm, critical thinking, and respect for the system you are part of.

Brent was one of those hires with just a pulse.

He was in his late 40s, tall, and talkative. On the surface, he was easygoing, even friendly to some of the other nurses. I wasn't so sure about him, though. He had the kind of personality that could disarm you if you weren't paying close attention. But it didn't take long for me to notice cracks beneath the surface.

I was the Charge Nurse one evening, holding down the medical office. As Charge, I couldn't leave to go interview inmates in other housing units—too many responsibilities and emergencies that might pop up in my own area. Brent was stationed in one of the Lockdown units when I needed his help.

An inmate had just come in, reporting to the Booking nurse that she was using prescription eye drops for a corneal ulcer. She had redness, severe pain, watering of the eye, and discharge for which antibiotic eye drops had been prescribed.. Before we called the on-call MD, we needed specific information. Where was she seen? By whom? What pharmacy filled the prescription? When was the last dose? Standard questions. Nurses could call the pharmacy to find out the directions for use, provided the patient signed a Release of Information. The on-call MD depended on us for this information before they could authorize a medication for a patient they'd never seen.

So I did what I had done countless times before—I picked up the phone and called the nurse working the inmate's Lockdown unit.

"Hey, Brent," I said, keeping a professional tone. "I need you to check in with the new booking in your unit—she reported using prescription eye drops. Please interview her to get the details."

His response blindsided me.

"What the fuck?!" he growled. "Why can't our doctor just write the damn order if another one already did?"

There was an edge in his voice that wasn't just irritation—it was hostility. Never in my career had I encountered hostility from a coworker. Nurses, in general, are patient, cooperative, and caring. No employer had provided any training for dealing with a hostile work environment.

I paused, unsure how to proceed. "We just need that information before we can call the MD. It's standard protocol. No doctor will order a medication for someone they have never seen without basic background information."

He exploded. "This is such bullshit! I'm not doing this! Why don't you come ask her yourself?"

I reminded him gently but firmly that I was Charge and couldn't leave. But he wasn't listening. He kept ranting, cursing, and throwing out insults like they were punctuation.

Eventually, he agreed to ask the inmate, but he made it clear he wasn't happy. I hung up, shaken.

And then I realized I'd forgotten one piece of critical info: the name of the clinic where the patient had been treated. So, reluctantly, I called back.

"What the fuck do you want now?!" Brent shouted into the phone before I could even speak.

I took a breath. "Just one more thing. Can you ask her where she was seen for the eye injury?"

He launched into another tirade, as if I were personally insulting him by doing my job. I tried to remain calm and professional, but I'll admit—I was rattled. Not just by his words, but by the sheer intensity of his anger over something so basic, so routine.

Again, he ranted. Again, I explained. Again, he grudgingly agreed to ask.

When I hung up, I stared at the receiver in disbelief. I wasn't used to being screamed at for doing my job.

That night, I couldn't shake the feeling that something was deeply wrong, not just with his behavior, but with the fact that someone like Brent could be trusted with independent nursing responsibilities in such a vulnerable population.

I sent a detailed email to our supervisor. She later told me she'd confronted him—and that he'd raised his voice at her, too. He eventually offered me a half-hearted apology, but not in a way that erased the sick feeling I had. The damage was done. From that point on, I found myself dreading shifts whenever I saw his name on the schedule. My trust in him was broken.

Weeks later, a second incident drove home just how dangerous trusting him could have been.

It was Brent's day off, and I was assigned to his usual dorm. Everything was quiet until I came across a diabetic patient scheduled for her nightly dose of insulin—55 units, as clearly ordered by the MD.

When I brought the syringe, the patient recoiled. "I don't take 55 units," she insisted. "Brent only gives me 15. Maybe 20 if I'm feeling high."

My stomach dropped. "Are you saying he doesn't follow the doctor's order?"

She nodded. "He gives me what I tell him I need."

I checked the diabetic flow sheet. Sure enough, Brent had charted the incorrect dose five times. What was worse, I noticed another nurse had followed suit, making it six charted, unauthorized doses in total.

This wasn't just a documentation error. This was a breakdown in patient safety. I refused to administer anything other than the dose ordered by the MD. So the patient ended up signing a refusal form declining the dose completely.

I immediately filed a Patient Safety Network problem report that got routed to the pharmacists and doctors. This wasn't something I could ignore. This wasn't just a policy violation – it was dangerous.

Brent was the kind of nurse who made my stomach knot when he walked in. Rude, incompetent, dangerous—he altered insulin doses without orders, documented lies, and snapped when asked to complete basic tasks. When leadership responded to my filing with only a verbal reminder, I felt sick. I knew full well he could retaliate to the Patient Safety report filing—or worse, even hurt a patient.

Later, I overheard our Supervisor talking to Brent in the hallway (which was safer than in her office). That alone spoke volumes.

"You need to follow MD orders, Brent."

He brushed it off. "She knows her insulin needs. She's alert and oriented. She tells me what she wants," he argued.

"She still needs a doctor's evaluation if the dose isn't right. You didn't call the doctor to change the order," she replied firmly.

He didn't seem to care. "Didn't think I had to," he shrugged.

There was no formal discipline, no accountability, no consequences. Management at the time decided a verbal reminder was enough. A reminder for a nurse who'd deliberately overridden medical orders, made up his own dosing, and documented it as if correct. This was criminal.

Brent eventually left Oakwood Medical. Good riddance. In the years following, leadership at Oakwood changed. New expectations, better oversight. Nurses like Brent wouldn't last a single shift under the current standards—and that gave me some hope. His departure felt like a storm cloud blowing off the building, and reaffirmed the moral weight nurses carry. But it left a lingering truth: inmates have no choice in their caregivers. We owe them better.

As for the patients? They were finally getting the care and respect they deserved.

Reflecting on these experiences now, I still feel a wave of anger and sadness. Not just for myself, but for the patients we were there to protect. At Oakwood, inmates don't get to choose their caregivers. That makes our integrity non-negotiable.

I still think about those nights. I think about how easily things could have gone wrong. About how professionalism isn't just about skill—it's about respect. For policies. For patients. For colleagues.

That's the kind of nurse I want to be – the respectful kind. That's the kind of nurse every patient should have.

> ***The wise man never says everything he thinks, he always thinks everything he says.***
>
> \- Aristotle

I Know That Name

Sitting at home, I heard a PBS narrator mention the surname Pleasant, and my heart startled—an inmate I knew had that surname. As the program unfolded with the extraordinary story of a trailblazing Black entrepreneur and abolitionist—I felt goosebumps. I thought of my inmate, of the legacies people quietly carry, unaware of the ancestors walking behind them. In jail, history and humanity weave together in unexpected ways.

One night, I was at home making dinner in the kitchen or getting ready to feed the cats (I can't remember which). In the background, hubby had his PBS channel on TV. He wasn't in the room listening; he just had it on as background noise. The television announcer was talking about something when suddenly, the name Pleasant caught my attention; I had known an Oakwood inmate with a similar last name. I stopped what I was doing to see what was on TV. The program was about notable people in California's history.

In the early 1800s, Mary Ellen Pleasant emerged as a remarkable figure, creating businesses and engaging in social activism amid the complex racial landscape of her time.

Born to uncertain parentage, Mary Ellen was believed to have a slave mother and a Hawaiian father. But her light skin allowed her to navigate society by passing as white, a strategy she used throughout her life. She married James Smith, a wealthy flour contractor. Together, they were involved in the Underground Railroad, a clandestine network helping enslaved people escape to freedom. Following Smith's passing, he left instructions and financial resources for her to continue their critical humanitarian work.

Around 1848, she entered a partnership with John James (J.J.) Pleasant. Though their marriage lacked official documentation, they continued the Underground Railroad's mission. J.J. traveled from

New Orleans to San Francisco to assess the city's potential as a destination for those seeking freedom. Mary Ellen left New Orleans for San Francisco by boat in 1852.

Pleasant arrived in San Francisco and quickly established herself in the city's competitive landscape. Passing as white, she took jobs running exclusive men's eating establishments.

She met many of the city's founders as she catered lavish meals. While waiting on tables, she paid attention to the discussions about financial agreements made over meals. At these establishments, she developed a keen business sense.

In time, she formed a financial partnership with Thomas Bell, a clerk at the Bank of California. By carefully leveraging information overheard during business discussions, they amassed a remarkable fortune of 30 million dollars by 1875, positioning Pleasant as a successful financier and civil rights advocate.

Mary Ellen didn't conceal her true race from other Black people who were brought to San Francisco by the Underground Railroad. Despite her financial success, Pleasant remained committed to supporting the Black community. She purchased multiple restaurants and employed recently arrived Underground Railroad refugees, helping them establish themselves in San Francisco. Many of these individuals became influential Black leaders in the city.

Pleasant's most significant civil rights achievement came in 1866, when she challenged racial discrimination. After being ejected from a city streetcar along with two other Black women, she pursued legal action. Her determination led to a California Supreme Court decision that outlawed segregation in San Francisco's public transportation system.

However, Pleasant's later life was marked by legal challenges that depleted her substantial wealth. By the time of her death in 1904, she had been reduced to poverty. In a posthumous recognition of her impact, San Francisco designated the smallest park in the city in her honor in 1974 – the Mary Ellen Pleasant Memorial Park, located at the southwest corner of Octavia and Bush streets, marked by eucalyptus trees she had planted outside her mansion.

One of our Oakwood ladies was a light-skinned African American woman in her mid-40s with a similar name and an amazing physical resemblance to the pictures of Mary Ellen Pleasant. I thought I would say something to her the next time I saw her.

One night during pill call a few weeks later, I whispered to her, "I watched a show about someone who might be related to you." She listened quietly as I described this amazing woman who tested racial boundaries, built significant wealth, and fought for civil rights. She didn't say anything in response to my description, but I could tell she began thinking about it. I never got to see her again to find out if she'd asked her family about a possible connection to Mary Ellen Pleasant.

We had other inmates related to famous people. Two people were cousins of famous country singers. Another inmate's relative created Disneyland, "the happiest place on Earth." One lady was related to a local politician; she was open about her family and her circumstances. They are just people trying to make it through this life, ones who happen to end up with us for a little while.

> ***In the end, it's not the years in your life that count. It's the life in your years.***
>
> \- Abraham Lincoln

Magical Power of Bright Pink Scrubs

After two draining weeks in the men's psychiatric unit, the tension seeped into my bones. One day, I wore bright pink scrubs on a whim. To my astonishment, the dorm softened—smiles appeared, tension eased, even pill call flowed smoothly. I learned that even small, intentional choices, with a little bit of hope, can transform a space.

Nursing school is a whirlwind of experiences. Rotations through Pediatrics, Medical/Surgical, dealing with medical illnesses and post-operative surgeries, Obstetrics to learn about Labor and Delivery, and Mental Health for exposure to a psychiatric facility. Each offers a glimpse into a different world of care.

While many of my classmates found new passions along the way, I always knew where I wanted to be: back at my beloved Medical Center on a Surgical unit. Still, I did the rotations, and even when I wasn't drawn to the specialties, I found them interesting, and I learned from them.

Over time, especially after starting work at Oakwood Medical, I found myself pulled into another world altogether, one I hadn't anticipated: mental health care inside a correctional facility. This is a growing population, because there are simply no other places for them to go.

I had just had a tough assignment lasting two weeks: the men's Special Management dorm. Having the same assignment for two weeks helps the nurses get to know the hundreds of inmates with whom we interact. I had worked in the women's unit before, but the men's was different. The men's dorm was a two-story open area, with no individual cells, just bunks, along with bars on the second floor to prevent anyone from jumping. A specially trained deputy was stationed there full-time—someone who could stay calm under pressure and act fast when they needed to de-escalate a situation.

Pill call was chaotic. It often felt like trying to run a medication pass in the middle of a storm. Meanwhile, pill call got stopped whenever additional deputies needed to respond to an altercation or a potential altercation in the dorm. Any small tension could halt the whole process.

"Pill call's delayed again," I said, half to myself, as I stood outside the dorm holding my med cart.

"Yeah," the nearest deputy said with a wry smile. "Happens whenever things get loud upstairs."

I gave him a look. "This dorm takes everything out of me."

He just chuckled softly. "It'll keep you humble, that's for sure."

As a matter of course, pill call for the men's Special Management dorm had the nurse situated outside of the dorm with their medication cart. One inmate at a time was allowed out. An officer was at the nurse's side at all times.

That particular night, an inmate had stepped up to me and told me quietly, "Ma'am, I need to see Mental Health. I'm feeling...homicidal."

He looked calm, almost too calm, and his words chilled me. I nodded and stepped away, alerting the deputy. Pill call stopped immediately.

Two deputies escorted him to a holding cell 30 feet away, close enough so deputies could watch him until Mental Health arrived. As soon as the door shut, he started kicking it. The loud, rhythmic thuds echoed through the hallway like a war drum.

"He'll be all right," one of the deputies said casually, wrapping waist chains around the inmate for his safety. "This isn't new for him."

But it wasn't normal to me. I tried to continue pill call, but my hands shook with each cap I popped. That night, his cries and kicks echoed in my thoughts long after I left work. I felt sad for him, but I also felt more respect for the deputies and MH staff who worked in Special Management for a living.

Even on my day off, I couldn't stop thinking about him. He had been taking his medications. He'd followed orders. And yet, he was in so much emotional pain that he didn't trust himself not to hurt someone. It hurt to realize that sometimes medication wasn't enough.

When I returned, I sought out a deputy I'd worked with before – the calm one who had spent 5 years in Acute Psych before coming to Oakwood. This particular deputy was so laid back and had a wonderful way with inmates who were upset/confused/having a hard time dealing with being in jail. I now felt even more respect for him since I had spent the last few days with the Special Management men.

"Hey," I said, catching him before he entered the unit. "Can I talk to you for a second?"

He nodded. "Sure, what's up?"

"That guy…from a couple of nights ago. The one who said he was homicidal? I've been thinking about him. It really got to me."

The deputy exhaled and leaned against the wall.

"Yeah. I remember him. It's tough. When I worked Acute Psych, we saw that kind of thing a lot. Doesn't make it easier, though. Just more familiar."

I looked at him, studying his calm demeanor.

"How do you do it?" I asked. "Stay grounded in all of this?"

"I remind myself," he said, "that even if I can't fix it, I can still be the calm in their storm. That counts for something."

I nodded, feeling a little lighter. "Well...it means a lot to see how you handle it. I have a lot of respect for the way you treat the inmates."

"Same to you," he said. "You keep showing up. That matters."

I headed out to pill call, trying to mentally prepare myself for any crazy, unexpected events that might happen at any time. After two draining weeks in the men's psychiatric unit, my spirit felt rubbed raw. The tension in that dorm seeped into my bones.

In the meantime, I had read that the color pink has been used in holding cells as it can help calm people down. So one morning, I pulled on bright pink scrubs—part rebellion, part psychological experiment. I figured, Why not try? I wanted to see if it helped with my interactions with these inmates.

When I entered the dorm dressed in my bright pink scrubs, a few inmates looked up. To my astonishment, the dorm softened. Men smiled, and the atmosphere transformed. Several inmates smiled and offered nice comments. Compliments floated through the air like gentle breezes. Even during pill call—a volatile hour—everything flowed with unexpected ease.

"Hey, nurse!" one called out, grinning. "You trying to bring some sunshine in here?"

Another chimed in: "Looking sharp in those scrubs!"

Their laughter wasn't mocking. It was warm and surprising. For a moment, the dorm felt lighter.

I smiled. "Just thought we could all use a little color."

Pill call went smoothly that evening. No lockdowns. No yelling. Just a few nods, a few small jokes, and calm faces—mine included.

As I pushed the empty cart back to Medical, I felt something settle in my chest: gratitude. Appreciation for the deputies who keep the dorms steady. Thankfulness for the MH team who show up every day for impossible tasks. Regard for the inmates who, even in pain, still smiled at pink scrubs. It was so nice to hear positive comments and to see smiling faces in this unit that had looked completely different two days prior.

That day, I realized how color, intention, and a little bit of hope can transform a space. Small things can make a difference. Along with maybe—just maybe—gratitude for being exactly where I was, in that moment.

An open mind will carry you forward.
Expand your mind and your long-term goals
- Elbert Hubbard

Helen, Quit It!

Helen, an exceptional mental health clinician, had a rare instinct for suffering—she saw the person beneath the symptoms. Inmates trusted her because she showed up with real humanity. So, when she confided that supervisors had told her to stop responding to "non-suicidal" needs, saying she was "raising expectations," my stomach turned. Watching her compassion punished by bureaucracy felt like witnessing something bright slowly dim.

Helen, a 60-something woman new to corrections, was one of my favorite Mental Health staff. She was more thorough in her interactions with the inmates than other MH staff. An exceptional Mental Health clinician, she had a gift—an instinct for suffering that let her see beneath symptoms into the heart of a person. Inmates adored her because she showed up for them, not just clinically but humanly.

As a result, deputies and inmates specifically asked for Helen. Deputies would refer to MH an inmate who can't stop crying or who insists he is having hallucinations. Often, when served by other MH staff, unsatisfied inmates would repeat their requests for MH support later the same day or night. Not so with the thorough care Helen provided. This led MH supervision to blame Helen for creating unrealistic expectations that made the rest of the MH team look bad. Her supervisor told her to only respond to suicidal inmates.

Here's how it went down. It was just after dinner one night, and the shift change buzz was still echoing down the hallway when Helen caught me by the elbow outside the room. She wore her usual soft blue cardigan over her county-issued badge and had that furrow between her brows that only showed up when something was really bothering her.

“Hey,” she said, lowering her voice. “Can I talk to you for a minute?”

“Of course,” I said, stepping aside from the flow of inmates being herded back to the housing units. “What’s going on?”

Helen exhaled slowly and looked around to make sure no one else was listening. “My supervisor told me I need to stop responding to every mental health request.”

I blinked. “Wait...what?”

She gave a little nod, lips pressed tight together. “Apparently, I’m too responsive. He said I need to save my energy for the serious cases—suicidal ideation only. That’s it. If someone’s just crying or thinks they're hallucinating, I’m supposed to ignore it unless a deputy insists it’s urgent.”

I felt my stomach turn. “That’s ridiculous. Just yesterday, one of the deputies told me they specifically asked for you. Said the guys calm down after you talk to them—stop putting in repeat slips all night long. You actually listen, Helen. That matters in here.”

She gave a sad little smile. “That’s what I thought, too. But my supervisor doesn’t see it that way. He said I’m making the rest of the team look bad. That when I see everyone, it ‘sets an unrealistic expectation’ for the inmates. His words.”

“Unrealistic expectation?” I scoffed. “Like what? That people in crisis deserve to be heard?”

Helen chuckled softly, but there was no joy in it. “I guess so. He told me, and I quote, ‘Helen, quit it. You’re not here to be Mother Teresa.’”

I shook my head in disbelief. “You’re doing what you're supposed to do. It’s mental health, not triage-only.”

She leaned in a little closer. “So I asked him, ‘Are you telling me I should ignore someone who’s clearly struggling, just because they aren’t actively suicidal?’ And he said, ‘If it’s not a suicide threat, it can wait. You’re wasting your time.’”

“Jesus.” I looked down the hall toward the pod. “You know how many guys here are just trying to hold it together for one more hour? One more night? And half the time they won’t say they’re suicidal, even if they are, because they don’t want to get stripped and thrown in a Ferguson gown.” Sometimes called a turtle suit, correctional facilities employed these thick quilted sleeveless gowns as a safety measure for inmates who posed a significant risk of self-harm or extreme disruptive behavior. The thickness prevented it from being rolled or folded into a noose. And Velcro fasteners were used in place of buttons, snaps, or belts. Hanging was a leading cause of death in jails.

Helen nodded, eyes shadowed. “I know. And the guys trust me. When I show up, they know I’m not there to punish or dismiss them.”

“So…what are you going to do?” I asked.

Helen straightened her shoulders and smoothed down her cardigan. “I’m going to do what I can. If I have time, I’m going out to see every referral I get. Quietly. Respectfully. But I’m not ignoring people just because they’re not screaming for help.”

A beat passed before I grinned. “That’s what I figured you’d say.”

She smiled back, this time with a little steel behind it. “They can write me up if they want. But if I can keep even one guy from spiraling deeper, that’s worth it.”

Watching Helen's spirit crumble under the weight of bureaucracy was like watching a flower get pressed under concrete. And with that, she turned and walked down the hallway toward the mental health office—shoulders squared, heart wide open.

YADA, YADA, YADA

- Seinfeld Episode 153

Reiki in Jail

I never expected to use Reiki at work, but one day a severely agitated inmate gave consent—and the calming effect was undeniable. I held my hands above her, letting the practice flow. Slowly, her breathing eased, her shoulders lowered, and the tremor in her voice faded. Deputies exchanged puzzled but grateful looks. In a place where calm is rare, the change felt almost sacred. Later, when she settled again from a distance as a result of me using remote Reiki, I understood: healing shows up in unlikely places—and in jail, you learn to use every tool available to you.

Every two years, nurses must complete at least 30 units of continuing education to renew their licenses. Over time, the classes have followed familiar patterns – cardiac care, respiratory, OB/GYN, trauma, wound management, chronic illness, and so on. Such are standard fare for the modern nurse. But in 2010, something different appeared on the course list: Basic Reiki.

Reiki, first practiced by Mikao Usui in Japan, is based on the idea that "qi" or "life force energy" can be guided to promote healing. Teachings claim that qi is physiological and can be manipulated to treat a condition or disease. Mainstream Western medicine largely dismisses it as pseudoscience, with clinical trials unable to confirm its efficacy. Still, I'd always been drawn to alternative approaches to healing. Curious and open-minded, I signed up.

Our instructor was a trained Reiki master who described Reiki as a gentle laying-on of hands—never a replacement for medical care, but a supportive tool. She explained its potential benefits: reduced stress, accelerated healing, emotional calm, release of anger, and the soothing of negative emotions.

That last part especially caught my attention. I had seen inmates, overwhelmed by emotion, punch concrete walls and break their hands after receiving bad news. If Reiki could help prevent that kind of pain, wasn't it worth a try?

She told us that over 800 hospitals in the U.S. had already incorporated Reiki use among their patients. I asked if it had ever been used in a jail. She blinked, smiled, and admitted, "Maybe not—this could be a first." I completed the two-day training with a fellow nurse from Oakwood's mental health unit. We were eager to return to work and try it out.

Not long after, I was the Charge Nurse one evening when a call came from the women's Special Management dorm. A patient was spiraling—anxious, agitated, and disrupting pill call. "Can I bring her to Medical?" the nurse asked. "Is the gurney available?" "Yes," I answered. "Bring her in."

Transporting a patient to Medical is no small task. It involves coordinating with the transportation deputy and requesting assistance when they are available. Then the deputies need to find a wheelchair to transport the patient. Once the transportation deputy arrives, the nurse will put her pill call medication cart away and accompany the deputy to Medical. The patient is transferred to the gurney and shackled. The nurse bringing the patient must give report about the patient to the nurses in Medical. Sometimes this process can take 30 minutes. If things work out, it can be as short as 15.

The patient seemed anxious and fidgety when she arrived in Medical. But just being alone in a room frequently calmed patients down. Dorms housed up to 60 inmates, and the constant noise and chaos could rattle anyone's nerves. My coworker nudged me: "Want to try Reiki?"

I took a deep breath and entered the room. I explained Reiki to the patient, a woman in her 40s. I asked for her consent to try this new, non-invasive approach. It was 8 p.m., so no psychiatrist on-call, meaning no quick fix through medication. She hesitated, then nodded her approval.

Reiki is about touching to heal. I remembered what our instructor had taught us: if touch might agitate someone, hover your hands above the person instead. I began by sending my intention that the patient receive the highest good as an outcome after my intervention. I could feel the channeling of energy to her. For good measure, I also sent Reiki energy to the gurney and the whole room.

Five minutes passed. She looked up. “I feel better,” she said. I rechecked her blood pressure. It was 10 points lower than when she'd first arrived in Medical. I encouraged her to rest. She stayed in the room, calm and quiet, for the next 90 minutes. Later, the nurse called to say she was ready to return the patient to her dorm. She and the deputy quietly wheeled her back to her dorm without incident.

I wasn’t sure if I believed in my Reiki skills just yet—but something had shifted. It seemed like she did calm down after my intervention. Little did I know I would need a different set of newly acquired Reiki skills for this patient soon!

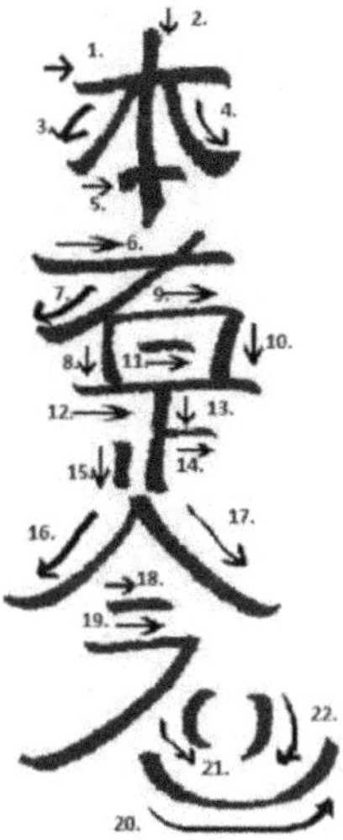

A few days later, the same patient was again in distress during pill call. But this time, we were overwhelmed in Medical—ER returns, man-downs, and altercations! The gurney was already occupied by another patient. But I remembered what we’d learned in the advanced class: remote Reiki.

I told the nurse I would try to use remote Reiki to calm the patient down this time. I brought up the patient’s information on my computer screen. I drew the Reiki symbol over the monitor and focused my energy.

Reiki is about energy. Symbols activate the process and allow the practitioner to receive the energy. Just five minutes of deep concentration, then back to the chaos around me.

I didn’t have time to check on the patient. But later that night, the nurse from Oakwood walked into Medical, grinning. “Right after I called you,” she said, “the patient just...settled down. We were shocked." She didn't know I'd sent Reiki. Neither did the deputy. But they all noticed the shift.

My new skills didn't just help the patient—they helped my coworker have a smoother shift, and maybe opened a door to a different kind of healing in an unlikely place. Reiki in jail. Who would've thought? But it worked.

> ***Positive energy knows no boundaries.***
>
> Lu Wei

Working with Unusual Staff

Some hires at Oakwood still make my eye twitch. There was Fran, who gave out sleep meds at breakfast, leaving inmates blissfully unaware but clinical schedules in shambles. There was Jean, whose communication was so unclear that deputies and inmates stared at her like she was speaking in riddles—and who charted wound care on the wrong body parts. And then Julie, whose leadership incompetence nearly imploded Mental Health entirely. These experiences underscored how dangerous poor hiring choices can be in a correctional environment.

Okay…it's time to talk about a few nurses hired to work at Oakwood Medical...

Hiring nurses to work in a jail setting can be difficult. The idea of working with criminals is scary. Knowing how vital it is to keep the Medical, Mental Health, and auxiliary staff safe keeps the custody staff coming back to work every day.

Most nurses I worked with were highly qualified, intelligent nurses with exceptional skills. When hiring, some nursing managers require recent acute care experience in a hospital, while other managers accept recent home care experience.

The most concerning hiring practice involves selecting candidates with a current nursing license, a pulse, and a pretty face rather than comprehensive professional competence. Three nurses in this category were unusual...

The first, Fran, was a pretty nurse in her mid-40s who claimed she had forensic nursing experience. Some of the nurses thought she was a racist, but we eventually decided she was indifferent to everyone. One day shift, Fran was assigned to a small unit of protected custody women who were seasoned inmates and had sophisticated styles of coping after years of being in custody.

This nurse was hired before our electronic medical records were implemented, so at the time we had to physically sign for each medication provided to patients. Morning pills given at 8 a.m. were typically for high blood pressure diabetes, or MH conditions, along with antibiotics, diuretics, and prenatal vitamins. Evening pills were typically mental health meds to aid in sleep, as well as cholesterol meds. Nurses administering meds in any given area knew which were generally given in the morning and which were usually given at night. (Note: a doctor ordered each medication to be given at a specific time.)

Fran demonstrated a fundamental misunderstanding of medication schedules. She administered sleep meds like Trazodone and Zyprexa at 8 a.m., a critical deviation from standard medical practices. She also administered more bedtime medications at 1 p.m. When the evening nurse came to administer meds at 8 p.m., she only found the 8 a.m. and 1 p.m. meds in the patient's cassettes.

Remarkably, inmates did not challenge these irregularities, viewing extended sleep as a quicker way to pass the time. The evening nurse asked the inmates what had happened earlier in the day. They laughed and said they thought it was strange, but they went along with it.

So the evening nurse began documenting multiple "incident reports" (one for every incorrect medication given). Despite clear evidence of systematic medication mismanagement, the initial response from her immediate supervisor was disappointing; they merely stated that "the situation" had been addressed. Fran continued to show up for shifts at Oakwood Medical. But a few weeks later, after another nurse manager dealt with her, she was no longer seen at Oakwood.

The second was Jean, a very pretty nurse from Asia who attended nursing school in the U.S. She had taken the NCLEX (the examination to qualify for a nursing license) and passed. Her previous employment was at a skilled nursing facility. She had severe English language limitations, which directly impacted her ability to communicate effectively in the high-stakes correctional healthcare environment. She was very friendly and did verbalize a few limited phrases in English. The other nurses expressed concerns about her communication skills with coworkers, deputies, and inmates, but they fell on deaf ears when it came to management.

One evening, her inability to understand English played out in a somewhat dramatic scene. Jean was assigned to women's Max North, single-cell dorms for inmates with mental health issues who had difficulty getting along with others. Some inmates there had histories of assaulting the deputies or each other.

During pill call one particular evening, Jean was standing outside the dorm where the severely mentally ill inmates were housed. Pill call was conducted through a slot in the main door. Inmates got out of their cells alone, one at a time.

Something went wrong. Two inmates who were out together began fighting. The two deputies at the control desk in the women's Max North unit dropped everything and ran into the Max North 2 dorm to de-escalate the fight.

The heavy metal door locked behind them. They yelled at Jean to push the button on the control panel to unlock the dorm door. Despite their frantic pleas, she had no idea what they were talking about.

The deputies inside Max North 2 called for backup on their radios. When backup deputies arrived at the outside door of women's Max North, they called out on the radio, "We are at the door – open the door!" Only then did they realize the deputies were locked inside the Max North 2 dorm!

They pounded on the door, trying to get Jean to push the other button to unlock the door to the unit, but she couldn't understand what they were saying. Many frantic minutes later, the officer at the Control Desk for Women's Max North building was able to override the door locks to let the deputies in to defuse the situation.

Even after this potentially dangerous event, Jean was not reprimanded. Meanwhile, deputies and inmates alike told me they had no idea what she was saying.

On one shift, I provided wound care for a patient; Jean had done the wound care the evening before.

The patient's wound was clearly on his face...but Jean had documented wound care to his foot.

The third nurse, Julie, was interviewing at Oakwood Mental Health for a senior management position. Julie wowed everyone with her skills and convinced the bosses she would be an asset to the team. Part of the interview process included determining if the candidate held advanced degrees; this is important when it comes to lawsuits. If the senior staff members are called into court, their credentials are an important part of their ability to provide expert testimony. One of the psychiatric nurses told me that Julie only held an Associate Degree in Nursing. This is a basic nursing degree. She was hired anyway.

After she was there for two years, with the expectation of her developing a competent Mental Health program, no policies or procedures had been written. There were complaints of mental health appointments not being scheduled. Julie also convinced one of the staff nurses to secretly record the nurses to find out why things weren't being done on time. The big bosses found out, and Julie and many of her staff nurses were let go from their jobs at Oakwood Mental Health. I was told by one of the remaining psychiatric nurses that Julie was a malignant narcissist. She had never been capable of developing a program.

One night, I got a "talking to" from a very mild-mannered deputy. I was standing in the open doorway leading to the outside of the Oakwood Medical lobby, trying to show a minimum-security inmate where to go to start taking a newly ordered medication. The patient seemed to have lots of questions about getting his new medication. At the same time, a nurse was providing wound care to a patient in Medical. The deputy couldn't be in both places at once to keep us safe. I was two doors away from the deputy. I heard the Medical deputy vigorously clicking the lock several times on the open door between us.

I came in to Medical, and the deputy yelled, "THERE IS NO WAY I CAN KEEP YOU SAFE WHEN YOU ARE OUT THERE!" He continued that he was working alone in Medical, and considering how dangerous the inmates in the minimum-security housing were since AB 109 had started sending inmates from prison back to the local jails when they violated their parole, he couldn't guarantee my safety. The deputies constantly watched how the inmates interacted with nurses. Some of them were quite sophisticated and had nothing to lose and would consider attacking a deputy or nurse if they thought it would earn them some points with their gang. Some of the inmates even provoked altercations to get "rolled up" to a particular dorm with their buddies.

His unusual "safety talk" reminded me that I needed to remember that my "patients" were inmates. This was the only time I was ever verbally chastised by a deputy.

> ***Always aim high, work hard, and care deeply about what you believe in.***
>
> \- Hillary Clinton

Leola Jay- Medical Records Savant

Leola was our quiet superhero. In the chaos of transitioning from paper to electronic records, she stood like a lighthouse—steady, glowing, unshakable. Lost detox form? She found it in minutes. Misplaced lower bunk order? Already in her hand. She held the medical unit together with grace, never demanding recognition. Her steady presence held our fragile system together. People like her are rarely celebrated, but are vital.

In the 16 years I worked at Oakwood Medical, two different electronic medical record (EMR) systems were rolled out. Each time, it felt like learning to navigate a new world. What had once been a room full of paper charts became a strange hybrid—half digital, half old-school paper. The change was chaotic. There were paper documents to notify DOC about patients who were detoxing from alcohol, patients who had a doctor's order for an ace wrap, patients who had an order for a lower bunk, etc. Piles of documents waiting to be scanned often grew like weeds in the corners of the Medical Records office. Processing these was a monumental task.

And in the middle of it all stood Leola Jay.

Leola had already been working at Oakwood for years when I started. She had this calm, grounded presence, like a lighthouse in the storm of paperwork and technology glitches.

She had been there through the change from paper medical charts to hybrid paper/electronic charts. Leola had a sixth sense when it came to finding lost paperwork. No matter how busy she was, she would drop everything to look for a particular document someone needed. There was a system in Medical Records to locate documents that awaited scanning by the staff. It seemed like a foreign language to the untrained ear. But Leola knew the system and could always be counted on to find "lost" documents.

“Where’s that lower bunk order for Jackson in M4?” a sergeant once barked, half out of breath as he stood in the doorway. His brow was furrowed, voice sharp with urgency. “DOC is on my back about it.”

I was already flipping through folders, my heart starting to race. That paper had come through earlier, but it hadn’t been scanned yet. I could picture it—a single sheet, hand-signed by Dr. Patel—but it had seemingly vanished into the void.

Leola didn’t even look up from her monitor. “Green tabbed folder, middle shelf, third slot from the left,” she said, calm as ever.

I blinked. “How do you—”

“Go ahead. It’s there,” she said with a smile, still typing.

Sure enough, I found the exact document right where she said it would be. When I handed it off to the sergeant, his demeanor shifted from frustrated to mildly impressed. “Guess you’ve got your own Oracle in here,” he muttered before heading off.

That’s how it always was with Leola. She had this uncanny ability to remember not just where documents were physically located, but the story behind them. “Oh, that was the day it snowed and the delivery truck was late,” she’d say. “That form came in folded with an ace wrap order from Unit 5.”

It wasn’t just memory. It was intuition. A sixth sense. And above all, a heart-centered way of being.

One night, the scanner jammed, and our stack of urgent documents was reaching a critical height. I sat at my desk, rubbing my temples.

“I don’t know how we’re going to get all this done,” I muttered. “They’re going to start yelling again in 10 minutes.”

Leola stood up from her desk and walked over with a mug of tea. “Let’s breathe first,” she said, placing the mug next to me. “Panicking never helped a printer.”

I laughed. “I wish they could hear you say that over in DOC.”

"They're just scared something will fall through the cracks. Same as us," she said. Then she rolled up her sleeves. "Come on, let's divide and conquer. I'll take Unit 2 through 4. You get 5 through 7."

Working with Leola always made things easier. She'd hum quietly while sorting papers, and somehow the air around her felt less tense. Whenever we were deep in a mess, Leola was the first to bring calm, not just with words, but with action.

"You're like some kind of wizard," I told her once after she pulled a detox intake form from what looked like a completely random box of miscellaneous copies.

She chuckled. "No magic. Just years of watching this place dance."

But I always thought there was a kind of magic to her. A soft, quiet kind. The kind that didn't show up in policy manuals or training guides.

In a jail setting, where tension ran high and compassion was often in short supply, Leola Jay was a rare light. When she looked at you, it felt like a hug. Like someone had your back, no matter how loud the radios squawked or how high the paperwork piled.

I didn't just learn record-keeping from her. I learned what it meant to lead with heart.

> ***Data is like garbage. You'd better know what you are going to do with it before you collect it***
>
> \- Mark Twain

A Livestock Trailer and Hay

Seeing hay scattered down the hallway nearly made me think I was dreaming—until I heard a soft bleat and saw a miniature pony round the corner. A nonprofit had brought a petting zoo for the women in Special Management, and what followed was magic. Hardened faces softened, withdrawn women lit up with childlike joy, hands reaching out to touch goats, chickens, sheep. For an hour, trauma loosened its grip, and the dorm transformed. I saw smiles I'd never seen before. Healing, I realized, sometimes walks in on four legs.

One afternoon, as I turned into the staff parking lot at Oakwood, I immediately noticed a truck with a large livestock trailer parked off to the side. I did a double-take.

Is that what I think it is?

The sight pulled something from deep within me, memories of raising pigs and steers for 4-H with my family, years ago. That smell of sun-baked farm animals and hay. It made me smile.

Probably just a rancher pulling off the freeway to check on the animals, I thought as I grabbed my bag and headed inside—*nothing to do with us.*

I didn't give it another thought, at least not right away. I clocked in and began my shift, making my way toward the Special Management and high security dorms for diabetic checks. As I entered the building, I noticed something strange on the floor...

Hay. That was something I had never seen in jail, not in my 15 years at Oakwood. Actual pieces of hay. Right there on the otherwise clean concrete hallway floor.

I stopped and looked around. "Am I seeing things?" I said aloud, laughing to myself.

"Hey, what's with the hay?" I asked the deputy in the control booth.

She looked up from her monitor with a slight grin. "Oh, that? The petting zoo is here. They're out in the Special Management dorm."

I blinked. "Wait—what? A *petting zoo*? In the women's *Special Management dorm*?"

She nodded. "Yep. Brought in some animals for the ladies."

I lit up like a Christmas tree.

"I've got to see this," I said, barely containing my excitement. "I just need to check my diabetics first."

"Go for it," the deputy said. "You'll want to catch it before dinner. They're only here for about an hour."

I grabbed my diabetic kit and raced to the dorm, buzzing in at the door. As soon as I stepped inside, I could smell the unmistakable scent of hay and animals; sweet, earthy, and entirely out of place.

I turned the corner into the yard and froze.

There, in the sunlight, were a miniature pony, a small flock of chickens, a goat, a pig, and two fluffy sheep. Several of the women were sitting in folding chairs, holding baby chicks gently in their hands. Others were crouched near the pony, brushing its mane or speaking softly to it. A few deputies stood nearby, along with a couple of volunteers in matching shirts from the animal therapy group.

"Hey!" I said, waving at one of the deputies. "Mind if I hang out for a few minutes before I start diabetic call?"

"You feed the cats, right?" she asked.

"Yeah."

"Then by all means," she said with a grin. "Want me to stash your gear?"

"Please!"

He took my diabetic kit and locked it in an empty cell. I stepped outside into the yard.

The change in atmosphere was almost spiritual. These women, ladies I had known for years, who usually wandered the dorm with blank stares or huddled alone in the dayroom, were glowing. Literally glowing.

One woman, Carla, was sitting on a chair, cradling a baby chick in her hands like it was made of glass.

I knelt beside her. "Hi Carla," I said softly.

She looked up, her eyes bright and focused, more than I'd ever seen them.

"I named her Sunny," she whispered.

"Sunny, huh? She looks like she likes you."

Carla nodded. "She's warm. Her heart beats so fast. I never held anything this soft before."

Another woman nearby was brushing the goat's back, giggling with another inmate. They were talking about what they'd name him.

"Marshmallow!" one said.

"No, Buttercup," the other laughed.

"No way, that's a cow name!"

I caught myself laughing with them.

Across the yard, I noticed one of the most withdrawn women, Tamika, standing still, hand outstretched, as the pony nuzzled her palm. Her eyes were welling with tears. A volunteer stood nearby, quietly watching but not interrupting.

A deputy walked up beside me.

"You seeing this?" she asked.

"I can't believe it," I said. "These women. This is the most I've ever seen them engaged."

She nodded. "I don't think I've ever heard Carla speak more than a few words until today."

I stood there for nearly 20 minutes, completely absorbed. The tension, the emotional walls, the despair that often hung in this dorm like fog, it was all gone. Replaced with laughter. Curiosity. Connection.

Later, as I finally got back to diabetic call, I couldn't stop smiling.

Every patient I checked was still talking about the animals, even the next day.

"They let me hold a baby chick!"

"Did you see the pig? He made this snorting sound—it was hilarious."

"Can they come back next week?"

When I wrapped up pill call hours later, the chatter hadn't stopped.

That night, I tracked down who'd brought the animals. A nonprofit north of San Francisco ran the program. They volunteered to come to Oakwood once a month—summer months only—weather permitting. I was stunned at the effort it took: loading up livestock, driving an hour each way, supervising inside a secure facility, then heading home to unload again.

All for one hour. One hour that changed lives.

After that, I planned my schedule around it. I arrived early—unofficially, of course—just to soak it in. The deputies on the women's side would smile when they saw me.

"Back for your animal therapy fix?" one joked. "You know it," I said.

Sometimes, if there was an incident elsewhere, the visits were cut short. But when they happened, they were pure magic. Quiet, powerful, and transformative.

It was a glimpse of unleashed humanity in a place built to contain it. The effort of loading these animals into a trailer to bring them to

Oakwood to hang out for an hour, and then loading them back into the trailer and driving an hour to unload them again was astounding. I was grateful to the bosses at Oakwood for allowing this to happen. I wished the psychiatrists, psychologists, and other members of the Mental Health department could have been there to see their patients.

Even now, years later, the memory of that first visit—the hay, the pony, the look in Carla's eyes—stays with me.

> ***One small positive thought can change your whole day.***
>
> – Zig Zig

My Favorite Inmates

Some inmates carved permanent space in my heart—Atena with her tall, athletic grace and easy smiles; Davey with his soft voice and gentle, genuine "How are you today?" during every blood sugar check; Trina with her intelligence and elegance despite the weight of serious charges; and Mr. Lodges, whose poise and dignity radiated even in a jumpsuit. They reminded me that humanity thrives even in captivity, and that connection often grows in the most unexpected places.

Working at Oakwood Medical for 16 years was a remarkably rewarding experience. I interacted with a wide variety of people I would not have met if I had stayed working in homecare, hospitals, or hospice. Many inmates had alienated their family and friends, so they came to think of the Oakwood staff and their fellow inmates as family. Over the years – after many, many interactions with them – I had come to regard several inmates as my all-time favorites.

One of those special inmates was Atena. She first came to Oakwood in her twenties – an attractive young woman, 5'10", physically fit, and quite outspoken when she arrived. Over the next few days, she quieted down and was respectful to the staff and other inmates. I had no idea what landed her at Oakwood, and I didn't care. There was a rumor that she had been awarded a full-ride sports scholarship, but being sentenced to jail had put an end to that opportunity.

She would be incarcerated for a few months and be released, only to show up again at Oakwood a few months later. Over the years, we talked about medical issues. Sometimes she took medication. I watched over the course of 10 years as Atena came and went, eventually making her way to the maximum-security dorm. I didn't know the circumstances of the move and didn't ask.

One of her most endearing attributes was her ability to display a huge smile on her face. She also seemed to brag about other members of her family being in jail at the same time. No one else did that. She never alluded to her life outside of Oakwood. But Atena always seemed upbeat in jail. Now that I'm writing this story, I think about her and hope she is okay. I'll always remember you, Atena. If you find yourself reading this, remember "March forth." I trust that you are safe. I hope you are happy.

Another favorite inmate/patient was Davey, whom I mentioned in the chapter about diabetics in jail. The nurses saw him a lot. It took about 3 minutes to get the lancet, alcohol pad, computer, and glucometer ready to check his blood sugar and administer the prescribed insulin. Over the years, we had lots of quick conversations in those 3 minutes, about an array of topics.

I never volunteered any private information about my life to any of the inmates. The safety talks the deputies had given to the nurses reinforced the need to keep details about our lives private when working with the inmates. But Davey shared with me that he had kids that he enjoyed walking to and from school. Over the years, he would change his hairstyle; he would wear it back or grow it out. When he eventually started wearing glasses, I commented that now he looked like a college professor. He always smiled when he heard that compliment. I didn't hear about anyone visiting him at Oakwood. I always worried because he was a small guy, which can be challenging in jail. But I never saw any sign of injuries, so he knew how to stay out of trouble. There always seemed to be an underlying sense of sadness about him. Yet Davey was always respectful and polite with the custody and medical staff. He always started the blood sugar visit by asking, "How are you?" in the most sincere, genuine voice. It always made my day. Davey if you find yourself reading this (and you know who you are): I only told the "how diabetes affects the groin" lecture to one patient. I pray that you are safe. I hope you are happy.

Trina was another favorite inmate/patient of mine. She was a strikingly beautiful woman in her 40s. Her story had been publicized in the local newspaper, so I knew why she was there. She was in the maximum-security dorm, which became my favorite. Ask any of my coworkers. She was in the dorm for a long time while her case made its way through court. She was intelligent, kind, respectful, and friendly. She had an unmistakable sparkle in her eye and a smile every time I saw her.

All inmates receive a TB (tuberculosis) skin test when they are first incarcerated. Thereafter, an annual check is required. A small amount of tuberculin is injected under the skin, and the reaction is read after 48-72 hours.

The annual injection was given to Trina. Seventy-two hours later, the nurse "read" the result and told her it was negative. No follow-up was ordered.

I was assigned to that dorm the following night. Trina, accompanied by another inmate who'd been an RN before her arrest, came up to me and demanded that I "read" Trina's test reaction again.

The reaction was positive, which contradicted the note in her medical record. I sent an email to the provider who sees patients with positive TB tests, and ordered a chest x-ray as mandated by the protocol, along with an appointment to follow up. The provider determined that Trina had converted to a positive result, but without an active TB illness. TB germs were present, but they were latent.

Trina was eventually sentenced to some time in prison and left Oakwood. Trina, if you find yourself reading this, I hope you are well.

My next favorite patient was Mr. Lodges. I don't remember his first name; I always called him by his last. He was a very handsome young man in his 30s who had Type 1 diabetes, so the nurses saw him frequently. His blood sugars were in the 300 range when he arrived at Oakwood Medical. It took a while, but he got his blood sugars under control. He had an elegant and well-bred air about him. He was suave and debonair like Frank Sinatra, but he was also really cool like Snoop Dogg. He seemed so confident and relaxed when we saw him at Oakwood Medical. He always had a huge smile when he came for his blood sugar testing. He was notably soft-spoken and intelligent. I didn't learn much about him during the 3 minutes it took to check his blood sugar and administer insulin as ordered. But as he left medical, I always got the feeling I had just experienced interacting with a member of royalty. He was special like that. I only saw him during a couple of incarcerations, but he made a lasting impression.

In reflecting on these individuals—Atena, Davey, Trina, and Mr. Lodges—I'm reminded that the walls of Oakwood held far more than rules and routines. They held people—complex, flawed, hopeful, funny, tragic, resilient people. These men and women were more than their charges or medical charts. Each had a spirit that managed to shine through, even in the most confined and clinical circumstances. Working at Oakwood taught me that kindness isn't about grand gestures; sometimes, it's simply listening, remembering a name, or offering a genuine compliment.

The inmates who became my favorites didn't do anything particularly extraordinary. They showed up as themselves, and left a lasting impression. I don't know where they are now. I don't know if they're free or if they've found peace. But I carry them with me, in the same quiet way they carried their strength. These stories are a small tribute to the humanity I witnessed behind the fences and locked doors.

> ***Think and wonder. Wonder and think.***
> - Dr. Seuss

Deputies Get Injured Keeping Medical Staff Safe

During a routine doctor's appointment, tension erupted without warning. The inmate lunged for a deputy's keys, triggering a violent struggle. I watched with horror as Deputy Harris injured his shoulder—an injury that never healed, eventually forcing early retirement. Later, I sat alone in the break room thinking about how easily deputies put their bodies between us and harm. Their sacrifices were often invisible—but never small.

At Oakwood Medical, healthcare for inmates runs around the clock. Nurses staff Medical 24/7, while physicians are on-site Monday through Friday during standard clinic hours. After hours, one doctor takes call (stays available by phone) until 10 PM every night. Inmates submit sick call slips to request appointments, which are reviewed and prioritized according to urgency. On the day of their appointment, inmates are notified by the runner assigned to the minimum-security area. They wait in the Medical lobby until called for their visit.

The exam room itself is small and utilitarian—just a desk, an exam table, a sink, and some supply cabinets. For safety, the door remains open. A privacy screen offers some discretion, and a deputy is stationed in the hallway just outside the room.

Most appointments are uneventful. But one weekday afternoon, that calm was shattered as the inmate's voice could be heard over the doctor's. The inmate was getting angry.

"All right," said Dr. Levin, glancing over the inmate's chart. "You're here for follow-up on your shoulder pain?"

The inmate, Mr. R., nodded, his arms crossed. He didn't sit.

"Still bothering you?" the doctor asked, clicking his pen.

"I told y'all this three times already," Mr. R. snapped. "Ain't nothing changing 'cause y'all ain't doing nothing!"

"I understand you're frustrated," Dr. Levin said, keeping his tone steady. "But yelling isn't going to help me understand what's going on. Let's talk about what's changed since last week."

Mr. R.'s voice rose sharply. "You ain't listening to me! I ain't playing this game no more!"

Dr. Levin stepped back slightly, his demeanor cooling. "This appointment is over," he said firmly. He turned toward the open doorway and addressed the deputy standing in the hall. "Deputy Harris, I'm terminating the visit. He needs to leave."

Deputy Harris nodded and stepped closer. "Mr. R., let's go. Time to head out."

Mr. R. walked out slowly, his jaw tight and shoulders hunched. But just as he passed Harris, he lunged.

"Hey!" Harris barked, jerking sideways as Mr. R. grabbed at his duty belt, his hand aiming for the keys.

"Officer involved 415!" shouted the second deputy, already reaching for his radio.

Chaos erupted in the narrow hallway. Deputies wrestled Mr. R. to the ground as chairs in the lobby clattered. The medical staff stood frozen for a split second, stunned by the sudden burst of violence.

"Get his hands!" someone shouted.

"Watch his left—he's reaching!"

In less than a minute, backup arrived. Three more deputies flooded in, securing the inmate and pulling him to his feet in cuffs.

Dr. Levin, still shaken, backed against the wall. "He just—he tried to grab Harris's keys. It happened so fast."

The nurses and medical staff remained at a distance, whispering to each other in disbelief. One of them, Nurse Jaime, muttered, "I've never seen anything like that in Medical... He looked so calm at first."

Once the situation was under control, Mr. R. was placed in a holding cell. The deputies cleared the area and confirmed he had calmed down. Then, per protocol, the nursing staff were required to assess him for injuries.

"He's clear for now," said Nurse Jaime quietly, after finishing the assessment. "Nothing requiring stitches or hospital transport."

But it wasn't over.

Later that afternoon, Deputy Harris sat on a bench in the staff break room, cradling his right arm. "You good?" his partner asked.

Harris exhaled slowly. "My shoulder's jacked. I felt it pop when he yanked me sideways." He tried rotating his arm and winced. "Something's not right."

"You should get checked out."

He did. He was sent to the ER for imaging and follow-up, but despite physical therapy and time off, the shoulder never healed properly. After months of trying to recover, Harris, early 40s, fit, respected by everyone, was forced to retire.

"He was one of the good ones," one of the nurses said when they heard the news. "Always calm, always fair. Treated inmates like people."

"Yeah," added another staff member. "Oakwood won't be the same without him."

The incident became a reminder of the risks deputies take every day, not just in the yard, but even in a medical room where most expect peace. Their vigilance protects not only the staff but the very structure that allows care to happen inside correctional walls.

> ***May your troubles be less and***
> ***your blessings be more***
>
> \- Irish Blessing

Service Dogs in Jail?

I almost choked on my coffee the day I saw a tiny dog trotting beside visitors during intake. The woman insisted it was a service animal, and custody let her through without verification. Jail rules flex strangely at times. A canine deputy later told me most contraband drugs came through the mail, not the public areas at all. I remembered an inmate who once wished her diabetic-alert dog could accompany her into custody. That longing stayed with me—sometimes the things people rely on most get stripped away the moment the doors close.

Let me tell you about a curious incident from my evening shift at Oakwood. I was just doing my usual routine – carrying a lab specimen to the West Gate and waiting for the courier to transport it to the lab. We didn't have an on-site lab, so we relied on these couriers to get our specimens processed after hours.

As I was walking through the lobby carrying lab specimens, something caught my eye. A group of visitors was heading toward the lockdown buildings, and – get this – there was a dog with them! Not a police dog, not a trained canine deputy, but just a scruffy little thing wandering around in the grass, off-leash, doing what dogs do best – sniffing everything in sight.

I'd seen drug-sniffing dogs inside before, but never a random dog with visitors. Curiosity got the better of me, so I struck up a conversation with one of the canine deputies. He had an interesting story to share about drug detection in the facility...

"Guess where we find the most drugs?" he asked me with a knowing smile. When I shrugged, he revealed something surprising - the mailroom. People tried to smuggle drugs into the jail by sending them on cards and letters. Inmates had a crafty method of getting high:

they'd tear tiny pieces of paper and pop them right into their mouths. The catch? The sender had to use a return address, which meant if drugs were found, the mail was confiscated and traced to the sender, who would be arrested.

Back to the mysterious dog. When I asked about this seemingly random canine, the deputy at West Gate told me the visitor insisted it was a "service dog." Interestingly, they had no paperwork to back up this claim. The deputy called his sergeant, who surprisingly gave the okay for the dog to enter.

We both stood there, scratching our heads. It reminded me of a story from a few years back about a "brittle" diabetic inmate. Her blood sugar would bottom out to dangerously low levels and the deputies would find her collapsed on her cell floor.

She had told me about the service dog she had at home—a specially trained companion who could detect dangerous blood sugar changes—and how she wished her dog could have been with her during her time in jail.

The whole situation felt surreal – a potentially unauthorized service dog walking freely among inmate visitors with no official documentation. It was one of those moments that made you pause and wonder about the unexpected twists that can happen during a routine work shift behind bars.

And as a healthcare professional, I'm always intrigued by these small, strange encounters that break up the monotony of a typical evening. The world of medical and correctional facilities is never quite as predictable as you might think.

This little incident stuck with me – a reminder that every workday can bring its own unique story, its own moment of surprise. Just another evening at Oakwood, where the ordinary can quickly become extraordinary.

You can have it all. Just not all at once.
- Oprah Winfrey

PJ

PJ was the kind of nurse who made everyone feel seen. He could calm rage with a conversation and steady a unit with gentleness and empathy. His gentleness carried us through hard days. Years later, running into him while feeding the feral cats—still unchanged in kindness—I was reminded: some people are anchors. You don't realize how much steadiness they give you until you lose it.

PJ started at Oakwood in his late 20s. He was one of the most genuinely compassionate coworkers I've ever had. Back then, he worked the 3:00 to 11:30 p.m. shift and had two little kids at home. He had this calm, steady energy. It was like nothing could rattle him. After a few years, he switched to the overnight shift, from 11:00 p.m. to 7:00 a.m., and yet his demeanor remained unchanged. He brought the same grounded, thoughtful approach to every encounter.

Late one night, many years ago, an inmate came into the clinic, clearly agitated.

"This is the third time they messed up my meds," the man said, his voice rising. "You people don't care. I'm sick of this!"

PJ didn't flinch. Calmly, he looked up from the chart in his hand and said, "Okay. Let's take a breath. Sit down here a minute."

The inmate stood there, fuming.

"I'm serious," PJ continued, with quiet firmness. "Have a seat. You're right to be upset if something's wrong. Let's figure it out."

Reluctantly, the inmate sat.

PJ pulled up the chart and started asking questions. "You're supposed to get your blood pressure meds in the morning, right? Did you get them yesterday?"

"Yeah, but not today. They skipped it."

"I see. It looks like there was a delay in the med run. Hang on." He stepped into the back and came out a few minutes later with a solution in hand. "All right. I've got it taken care of. You'll get your dose tonight. I flagged your chart so it won't happen again."

The inmate looked surprised. "That's it?"

"That's it. But if it happens again, you come straight here and ask for me."

The tension dissolved. "Thanks, man."

"No problem. You take care of yourself."

This was PJ, every night. He didn't just treat injuries; he treated people. With respect. With presence. He never let an inmate walk away feeling dismissed or unheard. It didn't matter how tired he was or what was going on around him. He gave each person his full attention.

When PJ interacted with inmates, they got his full attention. He talked with them to explain procedures, listen to complaints, and provide care for injuries. He made a point of talking to them until they calmed down and understood what was happening: a new medication, a discontinued medication, a cancelled appointment, or whatever the complaint was about.

I saw his same caring approach with deputies and fellow nurses. If someone had a rough day, PJ was the one to quietly ask, "You good?" or drop a gentle, "Let me know if you need a minute," without making a big show of it.

Nearly 20 years have passed since those days. And after more than two years of dealing with COVID, which burned out so many in this line of work, I wasn't sure who I'd see when I returned to Oakwood recently to feed the feral cats.

But I was walking along the back path, calling softly to the cats, when I heard a familiar voice behind me.

"Well, if it isn't the cat whisperer..."

I turned around. “PJ!” I said, genuinely surprised and thrilled. “You’re still here?”

He smiled, a little older but still unmistakably him. “Still here. Night shift lifer, I guess.”

We chatted for a while, and I asked how things had been since COVID.

“Rough at times,” he admitted. “But you know...You keep showing up. People still need care. That part hasn’t changed.”

And he meant it. That’s just who PJ is.

Seeing him again reminded me that, even in the toughest environments, it’s people like him – steady, caring, kind, and fully present – who quietly carry the place on their shoulders.

> ***I'm writing a book.***
> ***I've got the page numbers done.***
> - Steven Wright

The Secret Powers of the Nurses in Booking

When a police officer handed me a traffic ticket and asked if I had any questions, I smiled sweetly and told him my Booking nurse friends would "say hi" next time he came through. The way his face shifted—sudden realization, tiny flicker of panic—was priceless. Booking nurses control jail entry, and their medical decisions can reroute officers to hours-long ER visits. It's a strange balance of power dynamics, never straightforward, one that the public never sees.

Early one morning after I had been working at Oakwood for 13 years, hubby and I planned to take a lost dog to the shelter. We had emailed all the neighbors to see if anyone had lost this sweet guy, but no one responded. We took two cars, one with the dog, and I drove alone because I wanted to attend a cat show nearby after we got the dog to the shelter. I had been to the shelter several times to take feral kittens we found at Oakwood for spay/neuter so I knew the routine. It was a busy morning. I had to go to work that afternoon.

We arrived near the shelter and made a U-turn to drive into the driveway on the other side of the street. All of a sudden, police car lights were on us! I slowly pulled into the parking lot, parked, and sat with my hands on my steering wheel (as I had read was the safest posture after being stopped by the police). I sat and waited; no one came to my window. I overheard voices and turned to see the police officer talking to hubby. I got out of my car and joined them.

When I approached, I overheard the police officer speaking sarcastically, "I can see the sign from here...it says 'No U-turn.'" In all of my years at Oakwood, I had never been treated with this level of disrespect. I got angrier and angrier. But I knew I couldn't start being obnoxious. I didn't have time to get arrested before I went to work in the afternoon! We tried to explain we didn't live near the shelter and had missed seeing the sign.

He continued with his arrogant tone, "But I can read the sign from here and we are further away than you were in your cars." I bit my tongue and kept quiet. But I was fuming! He ended up writing only one ticket for an illegal U-turn – for me. He let hubby off the hook. After he handed me my ticket he asked, "Do you have any questions?" It came to me in a second! I looked at his name tag and said, "Officer P.....?" He replied "Yes." I said, "Well, I'll have to tell my nurse friends in Booking to say 'Hi' when you come through!" He looked at me and began mumbling unintelligibly. He knew this meant having the Booking nurse check for injuries.

The thing is, when anyone from Law Enforcement brings someone to jail to be arrested, the prisoner must be healthy enough to be incarcerated. In our county, the first person you see is a nurse in Booking.

If the nurse sees evidence of illness or wounds, the interview stops and the nurse insists the patient be medically "cleared" before being arrested. The quickest way to do this is to have them seen in the ER.

Having to take someone who is arrested to the ER can be time-consuming. If there are serious emergencies when an officer arrives with their arrested individual, they may have to wait until staff is freed up to help them. In other words, a nurse in Booking can really mess up your shift.

I still remember that officer's name. I worked with a nurse with the same last name, so it was familiar to me. After all this, I made it to the cat show and then to work on time...without getting arrested.

> ***You can choose to not let little things upset you***
>
> \- Joel Osteen

Bringing the Scale to Pill Call

I brought a scale into the maximum-security dorm for routine checks, and soon everyone wanted a turn. Two pounds lost. One gained. A number that hadn't changed. In a place starved for good news, even that felt like hope. For a few quiet minutes, that little scale gave them something rare—control, pride, a small reason to stand taller.

Working as a nurse at Oakwood means mastering a delicate balance of clinical skill, adaptability, and human connection. Each shift is a mix of medical responsibility and building trust within the walls of a high-security facility.

Most of our time is spent face-to-face with our patients—inmates who rely on us for everything from assessments to a simple conversation. During the 3-11 p.m. shift, we handle evening pill call and various assessments. One of my favorite assignments was the max security women's dorm. Challenging? Absolutely. But deeply rewarding.

"You got everything this time?" Deputy Collins asked with a smirk one evening as I approached the dorm.

I grinned, double-checking my cart. "Medications, BP machine, dressings, insulin, TB supplies... and yes, the portable scale. I'm locked and loaded."

"Good," she nodded. "You know the drill. If you forget something, you're taking the whole show with you."

That was no exaggeration. Just to leave and return, I had to remove everything for safety: cart, BP machine, and supplies. It was a logistical nightmare, and it cut into the inmates' program time.

One week, several inmates came in with MD orders to be weighed weekly for four weeks. I brought the portable digital scale in for the first time, expecting a few participants. Instead, a small crowd began to gather, anxious to step on the scale. I cleared their requests with the deputy, knowing it would slow down pill call.

"Nurse, can I check my weight, too?" one woman asked with hopefulness.

I glanced at Collins. "Is it okay if I weigh a few extras? It'll slow down pill call a bit."

She raised an eyebrow, then shrugged. "As long as it stays calm, go ahead."

What started as a clinical task quickly turned into a moment of connection. The women were eager.

"Down two pounds!" one exclaimed, grinning ear to ear.

"I gained a pound," another frowned, then added, "Guess I need to cut back on those commissary honey buns."

Their responses varied, but the scale gave them something tangible, something personal. A number on a screen that either lifted their spirits or gave them a new goal. It became a quiet ritual. For the most part, they were pleased. The only other time they could be checked was at an MD appointment. Their reactions varied, but they appreciated the feedback. It got to the point where the inmates would ask when I was going to bring the portable scale to pill call.

"You bringing the scale today?" they'd ask as soon as I entered.

It amazed me every time—how such a simple act could light up their faces. In a place where control is tight and choices are few, that scale gave them a sense of pride. Women who rarely got good news celebrated small victories—two pounds lost, one pound gained, a stable weight during stress. That little scale became a strange, tender, unexpected ritual of connection and motivation.

And me? I never forgot the scale again.

> ***Happy people focus on what they have.***
> ***Unhappy people focus on what's missing.***
> - Dr. Oz

Crocodile Dundee Behind Bars

Dotty, one of our beloved feral cats, struggled badly during COVID when volunteers couldn't enter the jail. Deputy Zukas took it upon herself to capture Dotty so she could retire in a sanctuary. Watching her wrangle that furious cat with a handmade loop—earning a deep scratch she called "Dotty's tattoo"—made me laugh and tear up at the same time. People assume deputies are hardened. Many of them are soft-hearted warriors.

Oakwood Correctional Facility is home to a surprising variety of wildlife—egrets, herons, owls, squirrels, ducks, seagulls, geese, snakes, opossums, skunks, raccoons, and more. Years ago, the grounds also supported a large population of feral cats. As these cats aged, they were gradually trapped and relocated to a retirement facility where they could live out their days in peace. Among the staff, no one was more skilled or fearless in managing this task than Deputy Zukas. She alone had the courage and composure to handle the cats when they needed to be captured for vet visits or relocation.

When the COVID-19 pandemic struck, access to the facility was restricted, and volunteers were no longer allowed inside. This posed a serious problem for Dotty, a six-year-old feral cat born on the grounds and living behind the Administration building. Her cozy shelter, built with care by inmates, remained intact, but her food supply quickly dwindled. With no volunteers to feed her, Dotty's survival was at risk.

Deputy Zukas, ever resourceful and compassionate, took it upon herself to act. She researched the safest methods for capturing feral cats and purchased a leash, cleverly adapting it into a loop for safe restraint. Knowing Dotty had missed a few meals, she used food as a lure. Dotty approached cautiously, drawn by the promise of nourishment, but she sensed something was amiss.

Just as Deputy Zukas positioned the loop, Dotty exploded with feral intensity. She fought with all her might, resisting the restraint with a wild, untamed strength. Despite the struggle, the deputy managed to secure her in a carrier and quickly covered it to reduce her stress and stimulation.

In the scuffle, Dotty left a lasting mark on her rescuer—a scratch Deputy Zukas wryly refers to as "Dotty's tattoo." Thanks to Zukas' bravery and determination, Dotty was safely transported to a retirement facility, where she now thrives. Her rescue was only possible because of Deputy Zukas's fearless intervention and unwavering dedication.

> ***Life is a journey, not a destination***
>
> - Proverb

The Tale of the Tables

How Four Mobile Tables at Oakwood Took on a Life of Their Own

When new mobile charting tables arrived during our switch to an electronic system, we anticipated sleek efficiency and high-tech bedside charting. Instead, the tablets couldn't get a signal inside cells, workflows were chaotic, and nurses were drowning in new procedures. Within weeks, the tables became improvised counters, shoe-tying stations, and clutter collectors. Jail has a way of reshaping the grandest administrative ideas into practical absurdities.

A few years back, excitement buzzed through Oakwood Medical/Mental Health. After years of paper charts and handwritten notes, we were finally getting an electronic medical record system—an EMR. For most, it was uncharted territory. But for me, it felt like a homecoming. I had used a similar program during my time in Hospice, so I was eager to help and share what I knew.

This story isn't about the EMR. It's about the tables that were rented to make this new process more mobile. Nurses could take them into the cells if the patient was experiencing a medical issue and couldn't get up to see the nurse in Medical.

"This is going to change everything," I said one morning, rolling into the nurses' station with a smile.

"Or break everything," muttered Rachel, one of the night nurses, as she stared warily at the new login screen.

To help ease the transition, administration had rented four rolling tables to make the EMR system mobile. The idea was thoughtful: if a patient was too ill to walk to Medical, nurses could take the tablet and chart right at the bedside. We could never get a signal in the cells, and with the security restrictions, mobility was essential.

"They're lightweight, height-adjustable, and easy to clean," the IT tech explained during setup, beaming like he'd personally invented the tables. "You can take them straight into the dorms!"

We nodded, impressed. The tables looked slick—white surfaces, smooth wheels, and just enough room for a laptop and some notes. We imagined rolling into cells like high-tech superheroes, charting vitals in real-time.

But then...things got busy.

Learning the EMR was like trying to build an airplane mid-flight. Everyone was scrambling to log in, troubleshoot glitches, and figure out where the "Save" button was (and if it actually saved anything). The tablets that were supposed to go out on rounds quietly disappeared from our minds.

And the tables never made it out to the dorms.

One afternoon, a week into our EMR rollout, I was looking for a spare surface to lay out some med sheets. That's when I spotted one of the tables—sitting unused next to the Pyxis machine.

"Hey," I said to Sara, our pharmacist. "Is that one of the mobile tables?"

"Oh, that? Yeah. We kind of... borrowed it," she said sheepishly. "It holds the Pyxis laptop now. Works better than that rickety old stand."

"Huh," I said, glancing at the clutter. "Is that another one over there?"

"Oh yeah," she laughed. "That one's for overflow paperwork. You know, scribbled notes before you enter things into the EMR."

It didn't stop there.

Table #3 found a home in the hallway, used by staff to set down boxes of gloves and unopened supplies. Table #4 disappeared into the pharmacy entirely, hidden beneath a pile of manila folders, a half-used bag of cough drops, and someone's old water bottle.

No one even remembered the original mission.

"Weren't we supposed to take these into the cells?" I asked one morning while watching a nurse use a table to lean on as she tied her shoe.

"Yeah, but we can't get a signal in there anyway," she shrugged. "And honestly? It's just easier to write the vitals down and enter them later."

In our own way, we were adapting. The EMR changed how we worked, but not always how we'd expected. The mobile tables, meant to revolutionize bedside care, had quietly transformed into permanent fixtures—serving new, less glamorous, but undeniably useful roles.

It was a lesson in practicality: sometimes, even the best tools get repurposed by the real demands of the job.

I took a few pictures of them—evidence of our noble, well-intentioned furniture now living quiet lives as glorified side tables. They may not have fulfilled their original mission, but in a place like Oakwood, everything finds a purpose. Even a table.

> ***Kindness is the language which the deaf can hear and the blind can see.***
> *- Mark Twain*

Why Is He So Mean?

Deputy Clark was infamous—intimidating, curt, impossible to read, harsh, and unapproachable. I spent years assuming he just didn't like me. Then one night, I saw him crouched in the dark where several feral cats hang out, gently petting one of them. His voice softened as he spoke to her, his entire face shifting into a state of vulnerability. In that quiet moment, the armor fell away, and I saw the man beneath it—the one who cared deeply but struggled to show it.

There's one deputy at Oakwood who stands alone—literally and figuratively.

Deputy Clark is 6'5", built like a linebacker, and as handsome as a movie star. Add a jawline carved from granite and a wife who looks like she stepped out of a magazine, and you'd think he'd be walking sunshine. But no.

Clark has a reputation, and it's not for charm. He carries himself with the kind of presence that turns heads and tightens stomachs. His attitude? Equal parts powerful and bad-tempered.

"Watch it," he barked once, not even looking up as a nurse accidentally brushed past him in the hallway. "You see how wide these halls are? Use 'em."

We all rolled our eyes, but no one said anything. You didn't challenge Clark. Especially not in Medical, and definitely not in Lockdown. Even inmates didn't mess with him. They could feel it—he was a man who didn't bluff. That worked in our favor. We felt safer when he was on shift.

Still, working around him wasn't exactly...pleasant.

One time, I tried to be friendly.

"Morning, Deputy Clark," I chirped, trying to break the ice.

He looked at me—just looked—and then grunted, "Is it?"

That was the end of that conversation.

He wasn't rude to his fellow deputies; in fact, he joked around with them sometimes, even smiled—rare, but it happened. But with nurses? It was all clipped words, snarling growls, and cold stares. I used to joke quietly with coworkers that if anyone ever pushed him too far, he'd explode into a giant, green version of himself—Oakwood's own Incredible Hulk.

For years, I kept an eye out for just a flicker of warmth. Anything. But nothing ever came.

Until one night.

It was late, and I was finishing an overtime shift. The compound was quiet, shadows stretching long across the yard. It was dark and no one else was outside. I was walking back from the women's dorm, alone, my footsteps echoing faintly in the stillness.

That's when I saw him. He didn't see or hear me.

Deputy Clark. Standing near the old shed where the feral cats tended to hang out.

At first, I thought he was just patrolling, maybe checking something. But then I noticed he wasn't standing tall and stiff like usual. He was crouched down, back turned, completely unaware of me. I paused, letting my eyes adjust.

That's when I saw it.

He was petting one of the feral cats.

I blinked, stunned. Our cats didn't usually come near unless you're offering food, and even then, they were skittish. But this one—Missy, I think—was rubbing up against his leg, purring like an engine. He reached out and scratched behind her ears with the gentlest touch I'd ever seen from the man.

"You're not so tough, are you?" he murmured.

I barely breathed. His voice was soft. Not gruff, not barking orders. Just…human.

"You remind me of someone," he said to the cat. "Always acting like you didn't care, but you did. You just didn't know how to show it."

Missy purred louder, and he chuckled—chuckled—as she rolled on her back.

"Well, don't go tellin' anyone," he added, ruffling her fur. "Gotta keep my rep."

I stayed frozen in place, not wanting to interrupt. That moment felt sacred—like I was witnessing something I wasn't meant to see.

Eventually, he stood, gave Missy a final pat, and walked off into the dark, the tough-guy swagger slipping back into place like a uniform.

I never told him I'd seen it. Never told anyone that I'd finally seen a tiny sliver of his softer side. But after that night, I couldn't look at him the same way.

Behind all that armor, there was something else. Something real. Maybe even something broken.

I continued thinking of that moment, namely when he was barking orders or brushing past without a word. And I'd smile.

Because I knew better.

> ***You can't have a good day with a bad attitude, and you can't have a bad day with a good attitude.***
>
> - - Scott Hamilton

One of My All-Time Favorite Deputies

Deputy Sakar was a hurricane of personality—loud, charismatic, gorgeous, hilarious, and somehow both terrifying and deeply loved by the inmates. Her signature greeting, "Hey, crackhead!" carried more warmth than insult, and the inmates soaked it up like sunshine. She enforced rules with a sharp edge but balanced them with humor that dissolved tension before it became danger. When she retired, the entire facility felt dimmer. Some people bring light into even the darkest institutions; Sakar was one of those rare souls.

Deputy Sakar was a pistol. She was in her 40s, with striking features and a presence that turned heads—not just because she was beautiful, but because she carried herself with confidence and no-nonsense energy. She followed the rules like they were scripture, but somehow still managed to make people laugh. And her voice—Lord, that voice—was high-pitched, melodic, and carried like a trumpet through the halls of Oakwood. She had a pretty good rapport with the inmates. Her claim to fame? Calling everyone "Crackhead"! Whenever she used the term, it was always in a caring voice, and everyone knew she never used it as an insult.

You could hear her coming before you ever saw her.

"*Crackhead!*" she'd call out, her voice echoing down the corridor, half-singing, half-laughing.

"*What are you doin' over there—trying to dig a tunnel to freedom?*"

As for the inmate she was talking to? Nine times out of ten, he'd laugh.

"Just lookin' for treasure, Sakar!" he'd shout back, grinning.

"*Treasure?*" she'd reply, walking up with her hands on her hips. "Boy, the only thing you're gonna find out here is disappointment and bad choices!"

But she'd say it with a twinkle in her eye. She never talked down to them, never made them feel small. Even when she was correcting someone, it was with humor and, strangely enough, a kind of care. She wasn't soft, not by a long shot, but she had a way of letting people know she saw them as human beings.

She had nicknames for almost everyone.

"*Come on, Crackhead #3,*" she said once, clapping a guy on the shoulder as he shuffled to the chow line. "You walkin' like your shoes are on backward. Pick it up!"

"Yes, ma'am," he said, chuckling. "You gonna retire before me?"

"Retire? I'm just gettin' started! I'm gonna be here till they carry me out in a chair."

But she didn't stay that long.

She retired a couple of years before I did. Quietly, no fuss. One day, she was there, and the next, she was gone. Word spread quickly: Sakar had turned in her badge and said goodbye.

After that, Oakwood felt... dimmer. Like someone had turned the volume down on the whole place.

There was no more echo of her voice ringing out from across the yard. No more "*Crackhead!*" shouted with that weird mix of mockery and maternal concern. The inmates noticed, too.

"Man, I miss Sakar," one of them said to me one morning. "She was the only one who called me that and didn't make me mad."

"She meant it like it was your middle name," I said. "Not your whole identity."

He nodded. "Yeah. She was different."

She was. Loud, funny, sharp, and impossible to ignore—but underneath it all was a heart that understood how to deal with people without breaking them down. And when she left, Oakwood didn't just get quieter—it lost a little of its soul.

A smart person knows what to say.
A wise person knows whether or not to say it.
- - Bill Gates

Halloween Costume Competition

Halloween was never supposed to be special in jail—but that year, the women's minimum unit turned toilet paper, yarn scraps, and allowed materials into magic. The creativity was astonishing—and the laughter was contagious. Bodybuilders were flexing cleverly padded jumpsuits, brides got wrapped in flowing toilet-paper gowns, cotton-candy costumes were spun from ingenuity and laughter. Deputies stood by smiling—genuinely smiling—as the women walked their makeshift runway. In that moment, the dorm didn't feel like jail. It felt like community, creativity, and a reminder that celebration can exist even in confinement.

Halloween has always been one of my favorite times of the year. There's just something about the rituals—the decorations, the costumes, and even the candy—that brings everyone together. If you have kids, trick-or-treating is the perfect excuse to chat with neighbors you might only wave at the rest of the year. And even if you don't, just putting a spooky goblin on your lawn and sitting on the porch with a bucket of candy for eager trick-or-treaters can give you that warm, social connection that leaves everyone feeling happier, kinder, and healthier. Honestly, these little moments of community can be contagious.

Every year at work, I'd show up in my Halloween-themed scrubs and bring some small props— harmless fun, but technically contraband. I even had this oversized fake rat I loved using to give a good scare to big, unsuspecting male deputies and inmates. The reactions were priceless, and it was all in good fun. Nobody ever seemed to mind the bit of holiday silliness.

One Halloween, over in the women's minimum-security unit, everything somehow lined up perfectly to allow a little celebration—a costume competition for one of the trustee dorms. Supplies were obviously pretty limited, and no contraband was allowed this time. But these ladies got creative, brainstorming costume ideas and cracking up as they figured out what they could make with the materials they had on hand. There was plenty of laughter, and they managed to keep the mischief to a minimum so the fun could continue.

The costumes they came up with were so clever! There were bodybuilders flexing imaginary muscles, brides dressed in layers of toilet paper, and even gangsters giving their best tough-guy impressions. One of the favorites was a cotton candy costume made from whatever they could scrounge up. Some of the women got artsy with handmade paper hats, rabbit ears, and masks. We even managed a little trick-or-treating with a limited stash of candy from the commissary.

For a few short minutes, these women got to let loose, be creative, and forget where they were. The deputies on duty were kind enough to allow these inmates a short time for a better frame of mind. The atmosphere was magic—just a special night of laughter and imagination that left everyone feeling a bit lighter.

> ***The joy of life is becoming a person you are proud of.***
>
> \- Bill Orender

The Greatest MD in Jail

Dr. Lawrence was a force of nature—kind, brilliant, endlessly curious. He treated inmates with unmatched respect, like human beings, not case numbers. He remembered their names, their stories, the arc of their lives across years. He defended thorough care even when deputies grew impatient. Fluent in Spanish and fascinated by frogs, whales, and weather patterns, he brought a sense of wonder into the sterile corners of medicine. He listened deeply and advocated fearlessly. When he retired, the loss felt seismic. He was the physician who made jail healthcare humane.

I must include mention of my all-time favorite MD in my four decades of nursing: hands down, it was Dr. Lawrence.

Dr. L was a lifer at Oakwood—in other words, most of his career was spent practicing medicine behind bars. And he loved it. He had the spark of someone doing exactly what he was meant to do. You could see it in his eyes, which lit up every time he walked into the clinic. He knew many of the inmates by name—some he'd seen grow from troubled teens into weathered men.

"I remember when he first came in," Dr. L would say, nodding toward a patient waiting in line.

"He was barely 18. Thought he was invincible. Got into fights over comic books." He'd shake his head, half-smiling. "Now he's reading philosophy. Imagine that."

He knew all the deputies, nurses, clerks, and even the janitors, often stopping to ask about someone's mother or mention a book he thought they might enjoy.

"Hey Sandra," he once called across the corridor to one of the medical clerks, "I left that David Attenborough DVD on your desk. You have to see the part about the cuttlefish. Just stunning."

His care for the inmates—our patients—was always exemplary. Dr. L was a fixture at Oakwood, and he truly *lived* the mission of Custody Health Services. He treated everyone with respect, curiosity, and a quiet steadiness that made even the most anxious patient exhale just a bit.

One quiet evening, I was restocking supplies when he peeked into the med room with a glimmer in his eye.

"Do you know the difference between a frog and a toad?" he asked, holding up a small book on amphibians.

"Uh... frogs are slimier?" I offered.

He chuckled. "Not exactly. Frogs generally have smooth, moist skin and longer legs—they're jumpers, and live near water. Toads? Dry, bumpy skin and short legs—they prefer to crawl or hop. Frogs have an athletic body. Toads have a squatty shape. And their eggs? Completely different." He opened the book and pointed to a photo like a proud teacher.

That night turned into an impromptu zoology lesson. From there, it became a running joke between us. He started calling me his "field assistant." Soon I began taking photos of lizards and spiders around my yard and bringing them in.

"Look at this one," I said one day, zooming in on a bright green anole basking on my fence.

Dr. L leaned in, squinting. "*Anolis carolinensis*! Gorgeous. Look at the dewlap—see that red throat fan? That's a male. He's showing off."

He wasn't just a walking field guide—he was a born enthusiast. When I told him about the red-winged blackbirds in my backyard, his whole face lit up. "Agelaius phoeniceus," he said, like he was greeting an old friend. Then came a delightful stream of facts and stories about the species.

"Did you know they're one of the few bird species where the female sings, too? Most people don't know that. And their territorial displays—pure drama."

He could talk for hours about nature, but when it came time for clinic, his focus snapped back to medicine. He took his time with patients, often too much for the deputies' liking.

"Doc," a deputy grumbled one afternoon, "you've got five more guys in holding and we're already behind."

Dr. L didn't flinch. He turned calmly to the deputy and said, "I understand, but this patient has a heart murmur we haven't documented before. Would you like to explain to the captain why we missed it?" The deputy backed off.

He was fluent in Spanish, which was an absolute godsend when caring for our many Spanish-speaking patients.

"¿Dónde le duele exactamente?" he'd ask, tapping his own side to guide a nervous patient toward gesturing.

"Aqui" the inmate would respond, showing him the spot.

"Vamos a revisar su historial—puede ser una úlcera," he'd say gently, already pulling up the medical records.

During Dr. L's visits, you could hear him quoting studies out loud, sometimes even debating himself.

"There was a 2015 study in *The Lancet,*" he muttered once, scanning a chart. "Hmm. But that was based on a non-incarcerated population...Still, the data might translate..."

He never stopped caring. Never cut corners. Never let the walls of the facility limit his practice or his humanity. His dedication to providing excellent, evidence-based care to this complex, underserved population never wavered.

When he retired, we threw him a party at Oakwood—because that was his home. His wife and sons came, and we filled them in on the *other* side of Dr. L—the prison doctor who debated pharmacokinetics while admiring dragonflies.

"Wait," his wife laughed, "he was still talking about frogs at work?"

"Every chance he got," I said. "And we loved him for it."

He made Oakwood a little more bearable. A lot more interesting. And absolutely unforgettable.

> *The difference between school and life?*
> *In school, you're taught a lesson and then given a test.*
> *In life, you're given a test that teaches you a lesson.*
> - Tom Bodett

Dancing in Medical Records

Alex, a new records clerk, arrived in Medical Records like a burst of unexpected joy. He loved gardening, quirky jokes, and—most memorably—dancing. Soon we developed a ritual: each time I passed his office, we'd exchange a couple of goofy dance moves. These tiny moments of levity became lifelines during difficult shifts heavy with crisis. In a place where stress sits like a weight on your chest, a silly dance can feel like oxygen.

Medical Records isn't usually the first place you'd associate with joy. It's a back-office world of filing cabinets, manila folders, and the pulsating thrum of printers spitting out paperwork. But it's also the quiet engine that keeps the facility's healthcare system running. The staff there provides the critical service of maintaining medical records and locating documents relating to patient care.

Even after the rollout of our latest electronic medical record system, some parts of the charting process remained stubbornly paper-based. Mental Health notes, custody-related alerts, and special medical requests all had to be documented on paper—then hand-delivered, scanned, or hunted down, depending on the day.

Custody relied on these documents. They needed to know if an inmate was detoxing from alcohol, needed a lower bunk due to seizures, or had been approved for a cane, soft-sided sneakers, or an ace wrap. Without this information, medical care plans fell apart...and so did whole shifts.

I learned quickly that building a relationship with the Medical Records team could mean the difference between leaving on time or watching your overtime hours rack up (again).

One evening, while picking up a medical health file, I noticed a new face behind the counter.

"Hey there," I said, offering a smile as I stepped up to introduce myself. "You new?"

The young man looked up, surprised, then smiled. "Yeah—first week. I'm Alex."

"Well, welcome to Medical Records," I said, shifting my bag on my shoulder. "I'm nurse Nancy Smith. I pop in and out a lot, usually in a hurry, usually looking for something I lost track of."

He laughed. "So, basically like everyone else I've met this week."

I grinned. "You're catching on fast."

We chatted for a few more minutes. I learned Alex was a gardener, just getting his feet under him in the department. I told him about my husband's latest drought-busting project—connecting two 275-gallon water tanks to our rain gutters.

His eyes lit up. "Wait, you're harvesting rainwater? That's genius. I've got a tomato garden that's basically holding me emotionally hostage. I water it more than I hydrate myself."

"Then you totally need a setup like this," I said. "My husband's practically a mad scientist with PVC pipe."

We both laughed. Then I added, half-joking, "Though at this point, I'm thinking we need to do a rain dance or something. It's been bone-dry for too long."

Alex raised an eyebrow. "You know," he said slowly, "I think you might be onto something."

The next night, I came prepared—with a few choreographed moves I'd thrown together in the hallway between rounds. When I saw Alex behind the counter, I leaned in and said, "Are you ready?"

"For what?"

"Our rain dance. We've got to summon the water gods, remember?"

He burst out laughing. “You actually made one up?”

“Of course I did. Step, clap, spin, and jazz hands,” I demonstrated, entirely unbothered by the puzzled looks from a passing nurse.

To his credit, Alex didn’t hesitate. He stood up from his chair, cleared a space between the filing cabinets, and mimicked my silly moves.

It became a thing. If I were slammed and couldn't stop to chat, I’d call out, “Alex!,” while passing by and do a quick finger wiggle—the universal sign for rain dance time. Without fail, he’d stand up, do a spin, and add a dramatic clap.

One night, as I was passing through Medical Records with a stack of documents in one hand and plastic bottles of normal saline for dressings in the other, I caught his eye and gave the signal.

He jumped up, did a flawless two-step and a snap, then bowed deeply. I laughed out loud.

Another nurse, watching with raised eyebrows, whispered, “Do you guys rehearse that or something?”

“Only when the drought gets serious,” I said with a wink.

That brief, shared absurdity in the middle of a chaotic shift gave me more than a laugh—it gave me a connection. In a place where emotions run high and the work never ends, that little dance reminded me that joy can live even in the most mundane spaces. Everyone knows dancing is good for the soul.

And honestly? I’m pretty sure we got a few sprinkles the following week.

> ***To dance, put your hand on your heart and listen to the sound of your soul***
>
> \- Eugene Faccuito

The Trustees Go On Strike

When the plumbing failed in the trustee barracks, chaos rippled through the facility. All 120 trustees were uprooted and relocated. The next morning, they united in a full strike—no laundry, no kitchen support, no janitorial work, no call slips. Medical froze. Nothing happened. Even the inmates who usually helped me refused, whispering, "Miss, I can't, they'll retaliate." I realized then how much the jail relied on this invisible labor force, and how quickly everything unraveled without them.

The Oakwood Correctional Facility minimum-security section included two barracks that each housed 60 trustees. These were men deemed well-behaved, reliable, and healthy enough to be given jobs throughout both the minimum and lockdown units. They were essential to the daily operations of the jail. Without them, the place couldn't function. Trustees delivered meals, handled janitorial work, and swapped out dirty laundry. They were the grease in the wheels that kept Oakwood turning.

That is, until the plumbing broke.

The announcement came down during the middle of a shift: the trustees' barracks needed emergency plumbing repairs: pipes leaking, toilets backing up, showers unusable. Facilities had no choice, they said. Every trustee was to be reassigned to any available open bunk in the minimum housing area. No one consulted the trustees or prepared them for the move. Just a sudden decision followed by a scramble of belongings and bodies.

"They can't do this," one trustee was overheard saying as he hauled a plastic bin of clothes to his temporary bunk. "They treat us like damn cattle."

The dissatisfaction turned to anger. By evening, word had spread like wildfire through the trustee ranks: they were going on strike.

It was just after 6 p.m. when their strike started, and the effects began to show. After count was cleared, I was prepping paperwork in the Medical Unit when I noticed something strange.

"Where's Randy?" I asked one of the evening nurses. "He usually picks up the call list by now."

"He never came," she replied, frowning as she glanced toward the hallway. "No one did."

That was a red flag.

Every evening, the Medical Unit sent out invitations—call slips—for inmates scheduled to have wounds cleaned, blood pressure checks, and medication reviews. The assigned trustee always picked them up. Tonight, the pile sat untouched. The trustee never showed up.

Soon after, a group of diabetic inmates began filtering in on their own for their scheduled insulin checks. These men were regulars, their faces familiar, their medical bracelets giving them clearance without a formal invite. But even they looked uneasy.

"You guys hear about the strike?" one of them said while rolling up his sleeve. "Trustees are done. Not doing anything until they get put back in their barracks."

"What do you mean nothing?" I asked. "You mean...not even Medical?"

"Not even laundry," he said flatly. "We told 'em it's a bad idea. But they're pissed. Said they ain't working like dogs just to get shuffled around like they're nothing."

"Will you help out in here tonight?" I begged one of the diabetics, desperation edging my voice. "Just run call slips for us? Just for tonight?"

He looked at me like I'd asked him to turn himself in for something he hadn't done. He flatly refused, knowing that if he helped out, he might face retaliation...

"Nah, can't do that," he explained. "If we break rank, we're the next ones to get dumped in segregation or jumped by our own."

He was probably right.

As the Charge Nurse on duty, I had to endorse the disruption to Night Shift. But without the trustees, our hands were tied. We couldn't call for patients. Couldn't change dressings. Couldn't get clean linens. The entire Medical Unit froze. Tension hung in the air like static before a storm.

The deputy assigned to Medical, usually calm and unreadable, paced by the doorway, whispering into his radio. The deputies were on edge, waiting to see if the trustees would start a fight.

"You think they'll start a fight?" a new nurse whispered beside me.

"No," I replied, though I wasn't sure. "They don't want to fight. They want to be heard."

The deputies were tense. Radios crackled. Phones rang with quiet urgency. We were all waiting. For what, we didn't know. Retaliation? Negotiation? A longer shutdown?

I left the facility that night with my stomach twisted into a knot. I was off for the next few days, so I never heard exactly how it was resolved. Of course, in the long run, the plumbing was fixed, they returned to their dorms, and peace was duly restored.

But I still remember the silence of the unit, the absence of familiar trustee faces, and the strange sense of power that came from their absence. They didn't raise their voices or pick up weapons. They simply withheld their labor, and everything stopped.

> ***People who wonder whether the glass is half empty or half full are missing the point. The glass is REFILLABLE.***
>
> \- Simon Sinek

Dr. Bells

Dr. Bells, our dentist, worked with the gentle steadiness of someone who understood how poverty and trauma shape a person's mouth. Most of our inmates had never seen a dentist before. He treated them with patience, dignity, and meticulous care—fighting to get treatment approved, advocating for surgery when policy wouldn't allow it. After extractions, he walked patients to Medical himself to ensure they received pain medication. His compassion filled gaps that the system left wide open. His dedication to underserved patients was extraordinary.

These stories wouldn't be complete without one about Dr. Bells, the Dentist at Oakwood Correctional Facility. He manages a program in which he, with some help from other dentists, treats patients from both Oakwood and the downtown jail. In short, it is a busy program.

Inmates are given a toothbrush and toothpaste when they are first housed, but must purchase replacements on commissary if needed later. The Sheriff's Department forbids floss because of its potential use as a weapon.

Many inmates ask to see the dentist. For most of them, this is the only time they see one. Inmates will turn in a medical slip to request to see the dentist to assess particular problems. Visits will be scheduled according to the severity of the need. So someone having difficulty eating will be scheduled sooner than an inmate complaining of a tooth that "sometimes hurts."

Unlike state prisons, where inmates have access to services such as dentures and fillings, Oakwood services are limited in scope to infections, x-rays, and the extraction of teeth.

Obtaining a dental appointment starts by filling out a medical slip and handing it to a nurse at sick call. The nurse obtains a set of vital signs. If the vitals are stable, the nurse will quickly look into the mouth to do a cursory assessment of any acute problems, such as signs of infection/abscess or facial swelling. Many of these patients have not had access to routine dental care. They have often not learned good oral hygiene. Many mouths we look into look nothing like what we see in TV commercials. They are not pretty, and many have tooth decay, resulting in a foul breath odor. As a baseline, the patient must be able to open and close their mouth without difficulty.

If any symptoms exist, the nurse will notify the dentist. If the problem is urgent and identified during dental clinic hours, the nurse presents the patient assessment to the dentist at the end of clinic. No matter how busy Dr. Bells was, he always had time to listen to a nurse's assessment of a potential dental issue.

If a patient had an extraction procedure that ended after pill call, Dr. Bells would go out of his way to escort the patient to medical and request that a dose of pain medication be given immediately. He did not want the patient to suffer in pain until the next pill call, many hours later.

One evening, a good-looking young man in his 20s approached me. He covered his mouth as he began talking. He complained of difficulty eating. I asked him to elaborate on the problem. He dropped the hand covering his mouth, and smiled. He had a crooked smile because his jaw was broken. His lower jaw looked like an inverted V! He shared that he had gotten into a fight and had his jaw broken a few weeks before being arrested and brought to Oakwood. He had also missed a scheduled dental appointment to begin the process of repairing his jaw. His lower teeth did not align with his upper teeth. No wonder he was having difficulty eating!

I immediately notified the doctor. He got the patient in to Dental and had x-rays done. Dr. Bells pleaded this young man's case to the administration. At the time, the policy would not allow any surgery to be scheduled for an injury that had occurred before incarceration. Dr.

Bells let me know he had tried his best but there was nothing he could do. He met with the patient and explained why he could not be scheduled for surgery at Oakwood. The "system" decides who gets surgeries, he said. So the patient received a chopped diet for the remainder of his time at Oakwood. I never saw this patient again.

*   *   *   *

Dr. Bells always arrives at Oakwood with a smile and a "Good Morning" – or a "Good Afternoon" on weekends if he comes in to catch up on paperwork. On weekdays, he is gracious and welcoming when the inmates arrive in the office. Patients fill out a questionnaire to better understand their oral health. After their visits, Dr. Bells can be seen smiling, shaking their hands, and saying, "Take care. See you next time." After looking at thousands of mouths that have been neglected and possibly poorly nourished for many years, he still has a genuine and respectful manner with each patient. Any inmate who has seen Dr. Bells at Oakwood will agree. He is one of the best dentists they have known.

Dr. Bells is also available by phone after hours, until 10 pm every night, for emergencies. He promptly answers every "page," obtains the pertinent patient information, and, if needed, orders medications for the patient or has the patient transported to the ER.

I was at an appointment with my personal dentist, having my teeth cleaned by my dental hygienist, who had been there for many years. I told her the inmates were using string from tea bags as floss. My dental hygienist thought this was quite creative.

Well, when I had been working as a nurse at Oakwood for more than 10 years, an inmate came to Medical requesting to see a nurse. He had gotten a tea bag string stuck between two teeth, and now it really hurt. We could not have Dr. Bells see him as his schedule was full. He was sent to the ER to have the string removed and was started on antibiotics.

Dr. Bells's career was a masterpiece in the way he consistently provided crucial dental care to this underserved population. Dr. Bells was such an extraordinary professional that this short tribute, for everything he did to help so many inmates, is essential to include among these Jailhouse stories.

> ***Take time to enjoy the little things,***
> ***for one day you may look back and realize***
> ***they were the big things.***
>
> \- Robert Brault

A Doctor's Order I'll Never Forget

Performing a sterile urinary catheterization inside a jail cell felt like nursing in a parallel universe. A deputy held a flashlight because the cell had no proper lighting. I balanced sterile technique with the unpredictability of a carceral environment. As I inserted the catheter flawlessly on the first try, relief washed through me. I realized how adaptable correctional nurses must become. In the hospital, this would have been routine; in jail, it felt like threading a needle during an earthquake.

Oakwood Medical schedules doctor's appointments for inmates during regular Monday through Friday 8 am-5 pm business hours. Patients are seen for a variety of complaints. During the appointment, the doctor assesses whether the patient will need more follow-up to clarify a diagnosis. The doctor may order blood tests, a specialty appointment at my beloved Medical Center, blood pressure checks, etc.

One of the Special Management dorm inmates complained of feeling like she still needed to urinate after she finished urinating. The doctor wrote an order for the nurse to perform a Post Void Residual test to determine the quantity of urine left in the bladder, which can indicate problems like an infection in the kidney or an obstruction in the urethra. This test can be done via ultrasound. Another procedure to determine the quantity of urine left is for the nurse to insert a urinary catheter into the bladder and drain the remaining fluid. All nurses are trained to insert a catheter. We are trained using sterile techniques, usually at the bedside in a hospital or beside a gurney in the clinic. There is always a chance of infection when inserting a urinary catheter.

When I found out the doctor had ordered a Post Void Residual for one of the ladies, I tried to remain calm. A hospital or clinic setting is kept fairly clean; however, a jail cell is dark and not regularly sanitized.

First, I gathered my supplies. The procedure needs to be done right after the patient empties her bladder, so I needed to be ready to go when I got the call. I asked the patient to notify the deputy when she had urinated. I notified the deputy in the dorm to call Medical when the inmate let her know, so I could come perform the catheterization.

When the call came, I headed out to the dorm, going over the procedure in my mind as I approached. The deputy had to lock down the dorm. It took a few minutes to get everyone in their cells. A second deputy stood by while I catheterized the patient. The tiny window high on the wall of the cell did not provide much light. I depended on the deputy's flashlight to help me see what I was doing. As I prepared my supplies, I explained to the patient what I planned to do. I tried not to think about the old mattress and the less-than-sanitary environment. The patient was very understanding and friendly.

I gloved up and picked up the drape that hangs in the straight catheter container. It looked very tiny in this particular setting. I placed a large plastic pad under the patient to help make the field a little cleaner. I then said a prayer and began the procedure. Fortunately, I was successful on my first attempt; I saw the amber fluid draining into the collection container.

Breathing a sigh of relief, I finished up, cleaned off the patient, thanked her and the deputies, and went to document the results of the Post Void Residual procedure. My catheterization of a patient in a jail cell by the light of a flashlight was something I'd never anticipated in nursing school. I was thankful that everything worked out.

> ***Don't cry because it's over,***
> ***smile because it happened.***
>
> \- Dr. Suess

A New Year's Eve Surprise

On New Year's Eve, deputies found a trembling dog wandering near East Gate. Without hesitation, MH Staff and I scooped him up, wrapped him in blankets, and cared for him while calls were made to find a foster. In a year full of loss, chaos, and exhaustion, ending the night with a frightened little dog in my arms felt like a tiny miracle—a reminder that compassion isn't limited to human inmates.

New Year's Eve (NYE) at Oakwood could go one of two ways: quietly ordinary or unexpectedly chaotic. The facility usually echoed with the sound of firecrackers from nearby neighborhoods, starting before sunset and growing louder as the night wore on. One particular NYE brought a different kind of noise—a call from custody staff that led to a heartwarming and slightly chaotic rescue unlike anything I'd encountered in over 15 years on the job...

It was early evening. The phone rang in the Mental Health office. I picked it up, half expecting a typical holiday check-in or maybe an update on patient status.

"Hey, Nurse," said Deputy Morales from the East Gate. "You might want to come out here. We found a little dog wandering near the street—it looks lost. Figured you'd know what to do."

I blinked. "A dog? Not a raccoon or a hawk this time?"

He laughed. "Nope. This one's barking, not squawking."

I hung up and turned to my colleague, Helen, one of our seasoned Mental Health nurses. She was sipping tea and flipping through paperwork.

"Hey Helen," I said, trying to sound casual. "Wanna go on a little adventure?"

She raised an eyebrow. “What kind of adventure? Because if this shift goes sideways after I say yes, I’m blaming you.”

“Fair warning—it involves a stray dog.”

Her eyes lit up. “A dog? You had me at ‘hello.’ Let’s go.”

By now, the deputies were used to calling me about injured wildlife. Over the years, I'd even made a few after-work trips to animal ERs to drop off injured birds found on the facility. Anyway, before I approached her, Helen had been having a quiet night. (Note: Nurses NEVER use the “q”-word; it’s a guarantee that our shift will “fall apart” with emergencies.)

We bundled up and made our way across the campus. The wind carried the sounds of distant pops and crackles, adding to the surreal, holiday-night atmosphere.

When we arrived at the old East-side kennels—long unused since Oakwood’s more pastoral days—Deputy Morales met us at the gate, flashlight in hand.

“He’s back there,” he said, gesturing toward the last kennel. “Didn’t look aggressive, just scared. Poor guy ran right in here when we opened the gate.”

We approached quietly. In the back corner, barely visible in the shadows, was a small tan-and-white dog, trembling and pressed against the wall.

“Hey there, buddy,” I said softly, crouching down. “It’s okay. We’re here to help.”

Helen knelt beside me. “Oh, my heart. He’s terrified. Probably fireworks and being lost. Think he’s chipped?”

“We’ll have to check, but first let’s get him somewhere warm.” We managed to coax him close enough to scoop him up. He didn’t fight us, just buried his head in Helen’s arm, shaking.

Back at the Mental Health office, we wrapped him in a soft blanket and set him down on the floor. He immediately crawled under the nearest desk.

"Can't say I blame him," Helen said, crouching to look under the desk. "If I were 20 pounds and lost in a firecracker war zone, I'd be under there, too."

I chuckled. "Think you can take him home tonight? The shelter's closed until tomorrow."

Helen didn't hesitate. "Absolutely. My mom's been wanting a dog. Maybe this is the universe's way of sending her one."

"Just don't say it's been a "quiet" night," I warned, only half-joking. "You know how that jinx works."

She laughed. "Too late!"

The next morning, Helen took the pup to the local shelter to scan for a microchip—nothing came up. No chip. She named him "Boomer," in honor of the night he'd been found.

Later that week, we caught up over lunch in the staff breakroom. "So, how's Boomer?" I asked.

She sighed, smiling. "Sweet as can be, but his anxiety is through the roof. My mom tried, but he wouldn't settle. Poor guy needs more help than we can give."

"Did you bring him back to the shelter?"

"I did. They've got a foster lined up who specializes in scared pups. He's going to be fine."

"Good," I said, feeling that familiar blend of sadness and relief. "You gave him a chance. That's more than he had out on the street."

We both sat in silence for a moment, sipping coffee while the firecrackers of memory still echoed faintly in our minds.

Another night, another story in the ever-surprising saga of Oakwood. And this one, even with its trembles and barks, had a kind of magic only New Year's Eve could bring.

Every firework begins with one spark.
One little spark can make big things happen.

Be the spark that ignites others
to light up the world.

-- Lynne Noe

Male and Female Inmates Together in One Building

A plumbing emergency forced us to house women temporarily in a men's lockdown building—a logistical nightmare. Every step had to be coordinated to prevent any accidental cross-gender contact. Despite the strictness, the women treated their escorted walks to their temporary housing like field trips, marveling at trees and sky they rarely saw. The week was exhausting but strangely beautiful: barriers held, safety maintained, no incidents logged. When repairs were finished, the women returned to their renovated dorm—still buzzing from the odd adventure.

Once upon a time—not so long ago, but long enough that everyone involved now laughs about it—the Lockdown women's dorm needed serious repairs. Plumbing issues had reached a breaking point. Literally. Pipes were leaking behind the walls, creating a mess no one could ignore anymore.

At Custody Administration, a dozen staff members gathered around a whiteboard covered in arrows, dorm numbers, and question marks in search of a workable plan.

"All right," said Lieutenant Rivera, arms crossed, "we've got 60 women to relocate, and we're out of empty dorms in the women's wing."

A long silence followed. Finally, Sergeant Kim spoke up, "What if we consolidated the men in Building 7 lockdown from four dorms to three?"

"You want to put the Lockdown women in a men's Lockdown building?" another staffer asked, raising an eyebrow.

"It's either that or tents," Kim replied.

After a long pause, Rivera sighed. "All right. Make it work. But no surprises. I mean it."

*   *   *   *

Moving day arrived like a military operation. The women packed their things into plastic bins and sat in neat rows, waiting their turn.

Deputy Jones, clipboard in hand, called out names. "Gonzalez, Maria. Unit 3C."

Maria stood up, waist already chained, and offered a mock salute. "Reporting for duty, sir."

Jones chuckled. "Let's try not to flirt with anyone through the vents, yeah?"

"No promises," Maria winked.

As the women shuffled slowly across the facility—feet shackled, waist chained, arms restrained—they marveled at their surroundings. It had been years since many of them had seen anything beyond the concrete of their own enclosed patio.

"Look! Trees!" gasped Toni, her voice muffled behind the woman in front of her.

"No way! Flowers and grass," someone else whispered.

Another woman leaned over and whispered, "This is like a field trip. Just slower."

Even with the clinking of chains, the procession had the giddy energy of a school outing—if the school had razor wire and armed escorts.

When they arrived at the men's Lockdown building, eyes widened.

"You mean...we're right next door?" asked Jean, craning her neck toward the nearby dorms.

Deputy Rhodes gave her a look. "Yes. And no. Yes, you're next door. No, you're not gonna be seeing anyone. This ain't summer camp."

Inside the building, everything changed immediately. Custody staff began redrawing movement schedules. Recreation times had to be completely separated. Even passing glances between windows had to be accounted for.

At the nurses' station, Nurse Betty blinked at her chart. "Prenatal vitamins? In a men's unit?"

"Surprise," said her partner, Nurse Mattie. "And we're doing all the vitals and wound care in their dorm now. No transfers."

"Are we expecting pregnancies or preventing them?" Betty deadpanned.

"Let's just say we're ensuring zero opportunities," Mattie replied, already filling her cart.

Behind the scenes, staff coordination was intense. But even amid the seriousness, there was humor.

"I give it nine months before we get an inmate baby boom," joked a deputy in the briefing.

"No chance," someone else replied. "Between us, Medical, and Mental Health, we're running tighter security than Fort Knox."

And they were. Deputies monitored schedules with military precision. The women were kept completely separate from the men—no overlapping movements, no shared spaces, no exceptions.

Despite the novelty of the arrangement, things ran smoothly. The women adjusted, the staff adapted, and the building—against all odds—kept functioning.

After several weeks, the repairs to the original women's dorm were completed. Moving day came again, but this time without the giggling or sightseeing. The women, now used to their temporary quarters, packed up in quiet cooperation.

As Maria stepped out of the men's Lockdown unit, she looked over her shoulder. "Well, it was fun while it lasted."

"Define 'fun,'" Deputy Jones said dryly.

Back in their renovated dorm, the women were met with fresh paint, fixed plumbing, and working showers. The whole ordeal had gone off without incident—no drama, no safety breaches, and, despite the jokes, no pregnancies.

It became one of those legendary stories staff would retell during night shifts and trainings.

Remember the time we housed the women in the men's lockdown?

Oh yeah. And not one single disaster.

Just a lot of planning, a little bit of laughter—and a whole lot of trees.

> ***Expect the unexpected and be ready to zigzag through whatever comes your way***
>
> \- Coach Bear Bryant

One Wild Night After Another

Exhaustion and responsibility never let up that week. Flu swept the jail, and as Charge Nurse, I made the hard calls while people around me grew sicker—quarantines, swabs, lockdowns, and even an attempted escape. The air felt constantly braced for impact. By the end, I was bone-tired, waiting for the next call—because at Oakwood, calm is only a pause, never a promise.

I tell you—this was one of *those* weeks. The kind you don't forget. I was Charge Nurse, which meant I was involved in *everything*. Every decision, every crisis, every "Can you come take a look at this?" landed squarely on my shoulders.

Tuesday night exploded right out the gate.

We were fighting Influenza A, and it felt like we were losing ground by the hour. This was pre-COVID. The fevers kept coming, and the minimum-security dorm quickly became Ground Zero. When the MDs finally said, "Quarantine it," there was a collective groan from nursing.

Every time an inmate spiked a fever of 101.2°F, the order was the same:

"Nasopharyngeal swab." In plain English? Take a long, cruel-looking Q-tip and jam it up a nostril until it feels like you've reached their tonsils.

One inmate recoiled. "You gotta be kidding me."

"I wish I were," I said. "Trust me, I don't enjoy this either."

Even the toughest, most snarly inmates flinched. It felt like sanctioned torture.

With the minimum-security quarantine, nursing turned into room service at the Hilton—pill call, temperature checks, diabetic call—everything delivered door to door. Then the flu jumped to Lockdown.

Great. More room service. Now everyone—staff and inmates—was walking around in masks. And then, predictably, nurses started getting sick, too.

Later, I talked to a nurse at the Main Jail.

"No flu here," she said.

"What?" I snapped. "Nobody?"

"Nope."

I shook my head. Oakwood has r*ecirculated air. No open windows. At the Main Jail, the stale air just sits there.* So we wondered why it spread at Oakwood but not at the Main Jail.

Unlike at minimum, these guys were stuck in dorms with sick inmates and nowhere to go. The MDs didn't hesitate. "Swab them. Transfer the sick ones to the Infirmary."

So we gagged them with the nose swab and shipped them off to the Main Jail.

I transferred two inmates that Tuesday night.

At one point, I called the on-call MD: "The lockdown nurse needs to talk to you. We've got an inmate with a 101.2 fever"

"Swab and transfer," he said, cutting me off.

He didn't ask for a name. Or a medical history. Or symptoms.

Just: *Swab and transfer.*

By the time my shift was winding down, all I could think about was getting outside, breathing real air, and feeding the cats. I *needed* that quiet.

Then I walked out to the women's area.

And there was a cat, Sammie. Stuck. In a skunk trap.

“Oh no, sweetheart,” I whispered, dropping everything. She was terrified but unharmed. I carefully got her out, then snapped the trap shut so nothing else could wander in and get caught. My heart was pounding harder than it had all night.

The next day, I called Shirley, who worked in custody as support staff. “We need that trap gone.” So it was removed. I left Janet a message to double-check on Wednesday night. Thankfully, Sammie was fine.

I thought maybe that was the end of the chaos. It wasn’t. The call went out over the radio for all available officers to respond. This results in a facility lockdown. No movement for custody, mental health, or medical personnel.

Thursday night brought a fight in the gang dorm. One inmate ended up needing sutures at the ER. As I prepared his paperwork for transport to the Main Jail, I learned he’d recently been interviewed by a Gang Affiliation Classification CO.

The gangs have their *own* classification. Somewhere at Oakwood, there’s a wall covered in photos—faces arranged by rank and status within the gang—a very different kind of family tree.

I finished the paperwork, shaking my head. *As if this place wasn’t complicated enough.*

By Saturday, foolishly, I thought things might slow down.

I signed in at West Gate and started my usual quarter-mile walk to Medical. As I came in, I saw a guy in his 30s from the minimum-security—handcuffed, surrounded by COs.

One of the nurses leaned toward me. “He tried to jump.”

“To kill himself?” I asked automatically.

She shook her head. “No. To escape.”

That got my attention.

He'd been arrested Friday night for violating a restraining order against his ex-girlfriend. Oh—and he was loaded with meth. A *significant* amount.

Apparently, on Saturday, he decided he *had* to get back to her. So he jumped a fence. Not just any fence—Candlestick fencing. He cleared the inside straight, vertical fence topped with barbed wire, made it all the way down to the Administration building, and tried to get through the exit gate—the one with the teeth that lock together. That's when visitors waiting for minimum visits spotted him. They alerted West Gate. And then all hell broke loose.

Oakwood went into immediate lockdown—right after I'd walked in. Four nurses and the supervisor were stuck at West Gate, unable to move. No one went anywhere until 3:30 PM, when nursing staff were slowly released back to Medical.

The escapee ended up with a small laceration—nothing major. But his ER trip? I overheard Correctional Officers discussing their understanding of what had happened:

Code 1. One Correctional Officer (CO) with him. A chase car following with two COs carrying rifles. Rifles. Because there was concern about a possible ambush at the ER.

So there they went: three armed COs, rifles drawn, escorting a waist-and-leg-chained, methed-out inmate straight into the ER.

I stood there afterward, exhausted beyond words. "I need a nap," I muttered.

And now? I'm screening my calls on my day off—just in case a sick call comes in, and they try to rope me back in.

Because at Oakwood, calm is temporary and *normal* is a myth.

> ***'And that's the way it is'***
>
> - Walter Cronkite, newscaster

Facing Off with Custody

Two other encounters with deputies stay with me. One barked at an inmate for asking about her medication, cutting across my role. Later, I learned she was in the middle of a brutal divorce. The anger wasn't really about authority—it was heartbreak spilling sideways. Another promised to keep me safe while scrolling his phone. I refused to start diabetic call until he put it away. He erupted, then froze me out for years. Advocating for safety and respect was uncomfortable, but necessary. In jail, working with custody required courage, boundaries, and compassion—even when compassion wasn't returned.

Two experiences I had with custody staff were quite disconcerting. The first incident was with Correctional Officer Breaux, a beautiful woman passionate about her work. One evening, while I was administering medications to a group of women, one of the inmates had a question about one of her medications. I always love it when patients show interest in learning more about their health and the medications they are receiving. As I organized my thoughts to begin a quick explanation of her medication, Officer Breaux shouted, "This is pill call! You are not allowed to interrupt the nurse during pill call! If you have questions, you will wait until the end and then ask!"

I was shocked by this response! The inmates were acclimated to hearing officers raising their voices during their incarceration. But it was completely irresponsible for her to react this way here. There were no time constraints to meet, nor was the building on fire. As a nurse, I am trained to answer questions about medications for patients. Teaching is one of a nurse's most important functions. The inmate who asked the question never waited for an answer.

When pill call was completed, and the inmates were no longer nearby, I approached Officer Breaux, with whom I had always had a positive working relationship.

"If you ever interfere with pill call in that way again when an inmate asks for information about their medication, I will report you to your Sergeant!" I yelled. This bold and fearless outburst was not in my character.

Officer Breaux broke down in tears; she was going through a contentious divorce and was having difficulty dealing with life in general. She apologized, and I ended up consoling her during this challenging time in her life. I never had another episode like this in my time at Oakwood. The custody staff knew the nurses were there to provide medical support through emergency care, medications, and, yes, teaching.

The other incident involved a correctional officer talking on his cell phone. I was sitting inside the medical office, getting ready to check the blood sugar of diabetic inmates before dinner in a Lockdown dorm.

Officer Tanal was seated outside in the corridor where the inmates lined up to be checked. From my chair at the desk, I could see him on his cell phone.

"First man up," the officer announced, meaning that the first inmate to have their blood sugar checked could enter the office.

"I'll wait until you are off your phone to start checking the diabetics, Officer Tanal," I immediately replied.

"Oh, I can keep you safe while I am on my phone," he countered.

I peeked out the door and shook my head toward the inmates. They heard everything I had said to the officer and understood I was going to wait until he got off his phone to start checking their blood sugars.

A minute later, he had an enraged look on his face. He put his phone away and began having the inmates enter the office for blood sugar checks. Officer Tanel didn't speak to me for several years after that incident. I personally couldn't hold a grudge for that long.

Advice I was taught when I first began work at Oakwood: Never interact with an inmate if a deputy/officer is on their phone.

> ***The next choice is the most important choice.***
>
> \- George Wells

A Halloween Miracle

One night, while feeding the feral cats behind Oakwood, I whispered to the universe that I needed a miracle. Moments later, former coworkers appeared out of nowhere, wrapping me in laughter and memories. That same night, I dreamed of inmates I had worried about—each one safe, smiling, stable. Weeks later, in a grocery store, a former inmate confirmed that some of those very women were doing well. It felt like a quiet blessing.

I retired after working at Oakwood for 16 years, but continued to return intermittently as a visitor to be part of the team that fed the second generation of feral cats. One sneaky female cat who wasn't part of our colony came to have a couple of litters; that's where we got our second generation. We eventually caught, spayed, and vaccinated her before returning her to Oakwood. "Trap, Neuter, Return" (TNR) tends to work.

I was assigned to feed the cats on the evening of October 30th – as mentioned, one of my favorite times of the year. For some unknown reason, I had asked the Universe for a miracle earlier in the morning that same day. I was chatting with Deputy Vasquez at the East Gate longer than usual. She was one of my favorite deputies whom I hadn't seen for a while. This woman was so drop-dead gorgeous and intelligent that she could be Miss Universe. Instead, she worked at Oakwood. She wasn't just beautiful, she had a wonderful relationship with the inmates, respectful and even caring when possible. I would have missed my miracle had I not taken the time to chat.

Out of the corner of my eye, I noticed a familiar face. Chris, one of my favorite Mental Health people, cared deeply about the inmates. She took time with them, and they knew she cared. Seeing Chris qualified as a miracle because she was no longer assigned to work at Oakwood; she worked at the jail downtown. But there was a staffing shortage at Oakwood that night, and Chris had come to fill the need.

Catching up with Chris was wonderful. It had been a couple of years since I had last seen her. I said goodnight and headed out to feed the cats. Hanging out with her was memorable. I felt happy to have seen her.

A few years ago, I created an "inmate satisfaction survey" and tried to get Oakwood management to implement it. My request fell on deaf ears. But if the inmates could designate their favorite MH staff, Chris would be at the top of the list. She really loves her work. After I got home that night, I felt a warm glow after having connected with her again.

I fell asleep and, much to my surprise, had a dream about running into Chris at the local grocery store. It was just like seeing her at Oakwood. It felt like I had not seen her for a couple of years.

Then my dream took a bizarre turn, as I visualized three of my all-time favorite MH inmates. These were young inmates in their 20s with severe MH issues.

Those of us who cared about these women knew they were safe only when they were incarcerated. Once released, they were at risk of being on the receiving end of foul play. None of them had any support from their families.

In the dream, one inmate, Mara, thanked me for talking to her about the feral cats at Oakwood. Reciting the kitties' names always seemed to calm her down a little. Mara told me she'd been transferred to a state hospital, and the people were taking good care of her. I said to her, "Mara, I'm happy to hear you are in a good place."

Julie, another inmate, told me she was arrested on the streets for drugs and for missing a court date. Her abusive spouse was now in prison. "He can't hurt me anymore," she said.

“I’m so happy to hear he can’t bother you when you are released from jail,” I replied.

A third inmate, Rena, said she was still at Oakwood after I'd retired. She had the same old mischievous look in her eye. Rena frequently schemed to fake an illness to go to the ER, or stage an MH drama to go to the psych unit. I looked at her and said with a smile, “You need to behave yourself.” Rena smiled back.

I was in shock in this dream; these were women I had worried about into my retirement. I woke up the next morning hoping my dream had a ring of truth to it, insofar as they were safe and being cared for.

A month later, I was at the grocery store I had dreamed about, standing at the bakery ordering a World Wrestling Entertainment (WWE) birthday cake for my son. He was in his thirties, but he loved the WWE. I flipped through the catalog of cake decoration choices but didn't see the WWE one. The lady in the bakery approached me. I asked her about that decoration. She frowned and said, “We don’t have it anymore. But let me check in the back.” I was waiting in front of several other people when she came back around the corner with the WWE decoration.

I knew it was a miracle. Excited, I proceeded to order the cake. When I was done, I turned to leave, and the lady behind me with a little boy was very interested in what I had ordered. I explained to her that it was WWE.

Then the most amazing thing happened. The third woman in line looked at me, and I knew the face but could not remember the name. It was Ms. Evans, a former Oakwood inmate. When she reminded me of her name, I immediately remembered her. She said she initially thought I was one of the deputies, but realized I was a nurse. I remembered that she was always very kind and easy to get along with. She said she had been away from Oakwood for 6 years and had gotten her kids back. She looked good. She had also spoken with one of the other ladies she had been at Oakwood with and gathered that a lot had changed since she had been there.

I told her I had seen one of my favorite inmates, Atina, walking in town the previous year, but I couldn't stop to chat. Ms. Evans told me she had spoken with her recently, too, and she was also doing well. Meeting up with Ms. Evans meant so much to me. "Running into you at this bakery has really made my day. Thank you, Ms. Evans," I told her. Hearing she was doing well and had not been back to Oakwood warmed my heart.

> ***Life is the first gift, love is the second, and understanding the third.***
>
> \- Marge Piercy

I Guess It Never Ends

One evening, I watched Deputy V crouch beside a young mother drowning in grief over her child custody case. He didn't lecture or judge—he listened. She was deep in fear about losing her children, her voice cracking with the kind of pain you feel in your own chest. He offered gentle, thoughtful guidance. In a place built on punishment, witnessing that level of compassion cracked something open inside me. His empathy moved me deeply. Healing doesn't always come from clinicians. It appears wherever a human being chooses to be kind, and sometimes the people wearing badges carry more tenderness than anyone expects.

It was a month after I'd unexpectedly run into Ms. Evans at the bakery—one of those brief but soul-stirring reminders that the work we do at Oakwood stays with people long after they've walked out those gates.

It was just after the holidays, and I was headed back to Oakwood to feed the feral cats. The weekends were always quiet—no evening visits, no outside programs, just the soft hum of routine behind the fences. My visits were simple: check in with the deputy at the West Gate, show my ID and the bag of cat food, then make my way to the yard where the cats lingered, wary but waiting.

That night, as I stepped into the front lobby, I saw something I didn't expect—something I'll never forget...

Deputy V, who usually greeted me with a clipped nod and a quick "You're good," stood just outside the intake area, speaking softly with a young woman about child custody issues. He reminded her about how important it was to protect her children. She looked no older than her early 20s, her thin jacket hardly enough for the cold night air. The woman was being released from jail. In her hands, she clutched a manila envelope and a worn canvas bag. The air between them was thick with the weight of something real.

"I don't know what I'm supposed to do," she was saying, her voice barely above a whisper. "My mom won't let me see them. Says I need to prove I'm clean first."

Deputy V's voice was low and measured. "That's not the worst thing, you know. She's protecting your babies. And if you love them, you'll see that as a chance—not a punishment."

She blinked, fighting back tears.

He continued, "Look, custody stuff is tough, but it's not impossible. You start with what you can control. Keep going to your check-ins. Stay clean. Get work, even if it's just part-time. Show up. Every day. You do that, and people start to notice." His passion for this subject matter was evident.

Her voice cracked. "But what if I mess up again?"

"Then you start over," he said gently. "Just like you did today."

There was a long silence. I stood just inside the doorway, frozen in place, not wanting to intrude. It felt sacred, like stepping into a chapel mid-prayer.

"Thank you," she said finally, hugging the envelope close to her chest. "Nobody really talks to me like that."

He nodded. "Well, someone should."

She gave a faint smile and walked out into the night, her shoulders just a little straighter than before.

When the door shut behind her, I approached slowly, still a bit stunned. "Deputy V," I said, "I hope you know that what you just did...that was more than just doing your job."

He glanced at me and gave a modest shrug. "She needed someone to remind her she's still got a shot. That doesn't cost me anything."

"But it meant everything to her," I said. "I could feel it."

He looked at me, a little softer now. “People think this place is just about bars and cells. But sometimes it’s about moments. Five-minute windows where someone decides not to give up.”

I nodded, my throat tight.

“I was just here to feed cats tonight,” I said with a half-laugh, “but I think I got fed, too.”

He smiled and held the door open for me. “Well, miracles come in all shapes.”

As I walked out toward the cat yard, I thought about how I'd nearly missed that moment. If I’d arrived just five minutes later, it would’ve passed unnoticed. Forgotten.

But I hadn’t. And in witnessing it, I was reminded—once again—that at Oakwood, the work never really ends. Not when you’re leading with your heart as well as your head.

> ***Speak the truth from the heart, and the right people will help you reach your goal.***
> - Lynda Barry

I'm Back… for Just a Few Moments

A routine evening of feeding feral cats at Oakwood turned into an unexpected emotional homecoming when a broken gate allowed me brief access to the women's building where I once worked. With the help of understanding deputies, I walked familiar halls filled with powerful memories, joy, and gratitude. For just a few moments, I was back in my favorite place—reminded of how deeply it still lives in my heart.

One evening, just like so many others, I headed toward Oakwood to feed the feral cats. The routine was familiar and comforting. I gathered my stadium bag with cat food and water, my heart already softening in anticipation of the cats who would be waiting, and entered the West Gate. One of my favorite deputies was on duty.

"Well, hey there," he said with a smile as I gave him my driver's license, which he exchanged for a visitor's badge. He had checked the computer for my security clearance the night before.

"Evening," I replied, smiling back. Small kindnesses matter in places like this.

I made my way inside and stopped first by Administration to give one of my regular feline friends a snack. He looked up at me expectantly, tail flicking.

"I promise I'll be back with your wet food," I told him quietly. "I just have to take care of the cats by the women's area first." He seemed okay with that plan.

I approached the locked gate, which gave me access to the women's area. I stopped short. A sign hung there, stark and unmistakable:

GATE OUT OF ORDER.

My heart sank.

This had only happened once before, two months ago—the first time ever for me. Back then, I'd retraced my steps to West Gate, feeding another cat along the way, and explained the broken gate problem to the deputy. There had been no immediate solution. I'd ended up texting another deputy who was working that night, and without hesitation he'd replied, *"I've got it. I'll feed them for you."* Later, I emailed Administration about the broken gate and was given instructions on how to navigate around it. The gate was fixed by the next night I was scheduled to feed the cats.

But here we were again. I turned around and went back to West Gate, explaining the situation to the deputy on duty. I shared the workaround Administration had previously given me—waiting by the rolling gate and having Control open it.

His expression darkened as he considered it.

"Control won't know why you're off your usual route," he said slowly.

I nodded. "That's what worries me."

His face remained dark as he thought about the options. After a moment, he said, "What if you go directly to Women's Control?"

I hesitated. "You know the rule: volunteers come in through the men's side. I don't want to cause problems."

He didn't argue. Instead, he picked up the phone.

"Women's Control," he said calmly, explaining the situation. I held my breath. When he hung up, he looked at me and smiled.

"They said it's okay. You can come through."

I must have thanked him three times.

As I got into my car to drive around to the women's side, my heart started pounding hard. I hadn't been inside that building since I'd retired. My favorite building. So many memories. The place that held so much of my past.

I parked, grabbed my license and stadium bag, and walked up to Women's Control. The deputy there recognized me instantly.

"Oh my gosh—it's so good to see you," she said warmly.

"I can't believe I'm here," I admitted, laughing nervously.

In my excitement, I forgot to sign in. She gently reminded me, handed me a badge, and guided me through the metal detector and into the sallyport. The door was heavy, and when it shut behind me, the loud boom echoed.

That sound made my heart sing.

Once I passed through both doors around Control, I was standing in the hallway I had walked countless times before my retirement. To anyone else, it was just a jail hallway.

To me, it was memory layered upon memory—favorite inmates, crazy episodes we had together, faces, voices, laughter, heartbreak, resilience.

I paused and took a deep breath. No particular scent. Just air. Just presence.

In my mind, a symphony of angels played as I danced pas de bouree down the hall. I smiled at myself—*In my head only,* I reminded myself. *Otherwise, I'd be 5150'd for sure.*

As I approached the door that led back outside to feed the cats, I was still in awe that I was *inside* again. My security clearance had been initiated at the height of the COVID frenzy. Administration made it clear that after I gave the deputy my license and obtained a visitor's badge, I would be required to stay outside of all buildings when I was there to feed the cats.

And yet here I was.

The cats noticed immediately that I was coming from a different direction. They looked at me with mild suspicion, then recognition, then enthusiasm. They ate eagerly as I filled their bowls and refreshed their water.

When I headed back toward the building, there was a song in my heart. I felt a deep, almost indescribable joy—happiness born from memory, gratitude, and grace.

All because of a broken gate.

For just a few moments, I was back in my favorite place, wrapped in the echoes of a life I loved.

You unlock this door with the key of imagination
- The Twilight Zone

Secret Language of Jailhouse Nurses

After my retirement, I bumped into a few former coworkers, and instantly it was like stepping back into a world only we understood. We swapped stories and frustrations, along with inside jokes about disappearing emails, impossible medication schedules, and the absurdities that once shaped our days—dark humor mixed with shared trauma, rapid-fire shorthand, nods that carried years of meaning. It struck me then: correctional nurses form a family forged not by blood but by crisis, grit, resilience, and a thousand stories no one else could ever truly comprehend. These bonds don't disappear when the badge comes off.

In an attempt to explain the following unusual exchange to the untrained ear, a few words to clarify how this story started on one topic, then veered off in different directions. Consider traveling to a foreign country where no one speaks your language. In that context, meeting someone you can understand might just constitute the highlight of your trip.

After being retired for several years, running into two people who spoke the language of "nurses who work in jail" was an opportunity to share similar crazy experiences at maximum speed, in a rapid-fire exchange of information. That means hitting all the highlights in a matter of minutes. It all made sense at the time – like a homecoming.

One evening as I made my way across the yard toward the women's building, my favorite of all the units where I feed the feral cats, I spotted a familiar face walking toward me.

It was Dana, one of my all-time most esteemed former nurse coworkers. She was heading toward Medical, wearing that expression

I knew all too well: a mix of disbelief, exhaustion, and something bordering on amusement.

"Hey Nancy!" she called out. "Still feeding your feline friends?"

"You know it," I said, holding up my clear stadium bag stuffed full of cat food and treats. "Living the dream."

Dana laughed. "Some things never change."

"Some things better not," I replied. "How are *you* doing? How's it going in there?"

Dana rolled her eyes so hard I thought they might stick. "Oh my God, you wouldn't believe the mess we've got going on now."

"Try me," I said, leaning against the rail while the cats circled my ankles, meowing with increasing urgency.

To put the following conversation in context: many years ago, a decision was made to close the Oakwood pharmacy and send the pharmacists back to my beloved Medical Center. Instead of packing up doses daily, pharmacists would now pack several days' worth of meds into cassettes for each inmate patient, prepared from a computerized med dispenser. The nurses were in shock, struggling to make it through the day with no pharmacists. Soon medical management decided that small quantities of the meds most frequently prescribed to the inmates would be left in a controlled stock for the nurses in the old pharmacy space. The stock medications were eventually placed within the computerized med dispenser so that there would be a record of medicines administered.

Nursing management met with the nursing staff and described specific changes that would be necessary. The nurses were to bring the meds needed for pill call, then return all the unused medication at the end of their shift. This included both prescription and over-the-counter meds. They explained the difference between the pharmacist's role of dispensing ordered medications and the nurse's role of administering medications. No medication brought by a nurse was to be left in the units when the nurse left at the end of the shift.

Some of the nurses cut corners to avoid extra trips back to Medical for one or two medications by stockpiling, that is, hiding extra meds in the units.

My conversation with Dana continued...

"Okay," she said, lowering her voice and glancing around as if someone might overhear us out there in the open air. "So, you remember when they pulled the pharmacy out of here? Packed it up, shipped it and all the pharmacists back to the Medical Center?"

I nodded. "I remember the chaos. The nurses looked like deer in headlights."

"Exactly," Dana said. "So, the fix was that the most-used meds would be kept in the old pharmacy space for nurses to grab during their shift. But here's the catch—they were supposed to take only what they needed for pill call, then return anything unused at the end of the shift. Prescription, over-the-counter, all of it. The meds couldn't stay on the units."

I smirked. "In theory, anyway."

She gave me a sharp look. "Yeah. In theory. But in practice? Let me tell you, Nancy, it's become a damn Easter egg hunt. I've been finding drawers and cupboards stuffed with extra meds. Nurses are stashing them so they don't have to make another trip to Medical. We're talking allergy meds, blood pressure pills, even insulin vials just sitting around."

I raised an eyebrow. "Seriously? Insulin?"

"I kid you not," she said. "I started collecting them, bringing them back to the pharmacy, and documenting what I found. Figured if I stayed on top of it, maybe it wouldn't get worse."

I shook my head. "Let me guess. It got worse."

Dana sighed. "Of course it did. And then it got *weird.* One day I got called into the office—apparently, some money was missing, and it was supposedly tied to those hidden meds. Someone hinted *I* might be involved."

I frowned. "Wait—money?"

"Yeah, that's the thing. They never explained how, but you know how rumors grow legs around here. After that, I stopped picking up the meds. I figured, if I'm going to get blamed, I might as well stop trying to help."

"Smart," I said. "What did your supervisor say?"

"I emailed her. Repeatedly. Told her what was going on. Want to guess what happened?"

"Nothing?"

"Worse. She deleted all my emails. Like they never existed."

I blinked. "She *what*?"

"I tried to pull one up the other day and—poof. Gone. Every single one I sent her about the stockpiling issue."

Just then, a nurse in scrubs approached us, coming from the direction of Medical. Dana waved her over.

"This is Nancy," she said, introducing me. "She used to be at Medical. Now she's retired but still comes to feed the cats."

"Hi," the nurse said with a smile. "Nice to meet you. I'm Sandy."

Dana turned to me. "She actually just helped me out. I called down to Medical and asked if someone could pull a med for me—I'll go pick it up myself. That's the right way to handle it, not hide it in a drawer."

"Always good to see it done right," I said, reaching into my bag for a handful of kibble. The cats were now practically vibrating with anticipation.

As I scattered the food, something clicked in my memory. "You ever work in Max North?" I asked Sandy.

She nodded. "A couple of times, yeah."

"Did you ever get stuck inside when the deputies needed you to hit the button to let them out of the dorm in an emergency?"

Sandy's eyes widened. "Yes! That *totally* happened to me. I didn't know what the button did, and I was afraid it might open the wrong door. I just froze."

Dana and I both laughed.

"Same thing happened to Jean," I said. Deputies got stuck in the dorm and needed her to push the button to let them out. "She told me later the deputies were yelling at her through the door, and she just stood panicked with fear."

The nurse chuckled. "Yep, that was me, too. Afterwards, one of the deputies came back and walked me through what button to push if it ever happened again. It's always something in that place."

Speaking of Jean, Dana leaned in. "You know," she said, "I used to try and say 'hi' to her all the time, and she never said anything back. Just totally ignored me. I couldn't figure out what her deal was."

"And?" I asked.

"Well, one day Jean comes up to me, totally out of the blue, and says, 'Do you know why I never said hi to you?'"

I blinked. "What did you say?"

Dana told Jean, "Please, enlighten me! Then she tells me it's because I'm 'with' one of the male nurses she likes."

I burst out laughing. "She thought you were dating him?"

"Apparently. I told her, 'He's my *friend.* That's it.' And after that, she was totally nice to me. Like flipping a switch."

"Workplace drama never dies," I said, shaking my head.

The cats had finished their food and were now lounging in a loose circle around us, full and content. I gave them a few extra treats for their patience while we'd dished out the latest gossip.

As I zipped up my bag, I looked at Dana. "Same circus, different clowns?"

"Exactly," she said. "And I'm just trying to keep the monkeys from setting the tent on fire."

Smile today, tomorrow could be worse.
- Minion Quotes

An Unusual Field Trip

At the county morgue, death lay before us—a woman lost to a house fire; a lifelong smoker's lungs blackened like tar; and a young life ended by gang violence. Death is often sanitized in nursing, hidden behind curtains and protocols—but here it was laid bare, unfiltered. The room had the sharp scent of chemicals and a heavy, reverent silence. That day stripped nursing of its distance. It left me with the quiet truth that we are fragile, and how sacred the act of caring truly is.

Nursing is a profession that demands continuous learning. The ever-evolving landscape of medical technology, medications, and treatment options necessitates that nurses stay current to deliver the best possible care. As part of the license renewal process, nurses must complete a set number of continuing education hours every two years. There is an enormous volume of classes from which to choose.

Oakwood Medical specifically assigned Jenny, a dedicated Staff Developer, to seek out relevant courses tailored to our specific work environment—correctional healthcare. In a groundbreaking move, she told us she had arranged a unique, unconventional, extraordinary learning opportunity for nurses and custody staff in the last place anyone could imagine. I was intrigued. However, when she revealed the destination, intrigue turned to apprehension...

"We're going to the morgue," she said with a small, knowing smile.

The idea of spending time in a morgue was unsettling for many of us. I had dealt with death before, but always in the context of patient care—doing everything possible to prevent it— or, in hospice, to make it as comfortable as possible. This experience would be different. We would be standing face-to-face with the reality of mortality in a way most medical professionals never do.

As I prepared for this experience, I reflected on my time as a nurse's aide in the hospital. One moment in particular stood out – the first time I was assigned to transport a deceased patient to the morgue. Decades ago, the morgue was located in the hospital's basement. A nurse gave me directions and called ahead to inform them that I was en route. As I stepped out of the elevator, the dim lighting and eerie silence of the basement stood out in a stark contrast to the bright and active patient units I was accustomed to. I felt uneasy and overwhelmed with this task, but there was no turning back. Reaching the morgue, I pressed the security button to the entrance. The door buzzed, and with a deep breath, I slowly pushed the gurney inside. Just as I braced myself for what lay ahead, an unexpected sight momentarily distracted me: some of the morgue staff were casually sitting around eating food! Here I was, grappling with the solemnity of my task while they carried on with their routine. My surprise quickly faded as they noticed me and sprang into action. They guided my gurney to a specific enclosure, carefully transferred the body, and returned the empty gurney to me. It was a situation I would never forget – a distinct reminder of how different environments shape our perceptions of life and death.

The morning of our field trip, I arrived at the county morgue located in a separate building behind my beloved medical center. The air was thick with anticipation and unease as we awaited the educational experience that would unfold in this most unexpected of classrooms. A coroner greeted us and provided a brief orientation. Visitors were required to sign a document stating that we would maintain a professional and respectful demeanor at all times. The deceased deserved dignity, even in death.

Preparation for the morgue tour involved strict protocols. Participants were issued protective equipment, including masks to mitigate odors and paper gowns to cover our clothing. We donned the masks and paper gowns, our hearts pounding in our chests. Stepping into the lab, we were immediately met with the sharp scent of chemicals mingled with a faint, underlying odor of decay. The lab environment was carefully controlled, roped off eight feet from the bodies, providing a safe distance for observation while allowing the technicians to continue their critical work. The technicians were young and adorned with body art tattoos. Silver rings and studs highlighted their nose, lips, and ear piercings. Jet black hair accentuated their black gothic attire, which was worn under their lab coats.

The educational session presented three distinct case studies, each offering unique insights into forensic pathology and the complex circumstances surrounding human mortality.

The first body belonged to an elderly woman who had tragically perished in a house fire. Confined to a wheelchair, she had been home alone when flames consumed the mobile home she shared with her husband. He had only left for a few minutes to drive to the store to buy milk. The coroner explained that her body was so severely burned that performing a full autopsy would be exceedingly difficult. The sight of her charred remains was sobering. This case highlighted the unpredictability of life-threatening situations and the importance of fire safety.

Next, we were introduced to a man in his 60s found unresponsive in his truck with the engine running. The coroner carefully removed a lung and held it up for us to see. Years of smoking had ravaged the organ, leaving it blackened and deteriorated. The visual impact was profound—more powerful than any anti-smoking campaign. The examination continued, revealing a significant accumulation of adipose (fat) deposits in his abdomen and damage to his heart muscle. Blocked coronary arteries painted a clear picture of a lifetime of unhealthy habits.

At the far end of the room lay the final body, surrounded by more staff than the others. They advised us to keep our distance. The young man had been in his 20s, a former gang member attempting to turn his life around. He had moved away from his old neighborhood, into an older, quiet section of town, hoping for a fresh start out of gang life. But gang violence has a long reach. A drive-by shooter had taken his life as he stood in his front yard. The fatal gunshot wound to his temple told the story of a life cut short, full of unrealized potential. Several police detectives were present, their expressions unreadable as they observed the autopsy. The details of his case were not shared with us, but the weight of his loss was unmistakable. The local newspaper later ran a piece on his attempt to leave gang life behind—a tragic reminder of how difficult escape from that life can be.

As our time at the morgue concluded, we thanked the coroners for allowing us to witness their work firsthand. Walking out into the daylight, the world felt different. Our experience had been profound and somber. We had stepped into a space where life had already ended and where stories had reached their final chapter. The visual and emotional impact of the experience spoke volumes. There was no test to take after this field trip, no formal discussion to process what we had seen. But in the quiet moments afterward, I reflected. This was not just a lesson in anatomy or pathology; it was a life lesson in choices, the fragility of our existence, and the complex circumstances surrounding mortality.

This extraordinary educational experience exemplified the innovative approaches healthcare institutions can employ to support ongoing professional development, pushing the boundaries of traditional learning methods while maintaining the utmost respect for human dignity.

Some experiences change you. This was one of them.

> ***Recognize what you have inside you.***
>
> \- Eric Pulier

Conclusion

Sixteen years at Oakwood left me with a heart full of memories mixed with grief, awe, and love. I entered as a nurse; I left changed—shaped by inmates who trusted me, deputies who stood guard, coworkers who carried me through impossible shifts. I witnessed cruelty and resilience, horror and humor, despair and fierce compassion. Writing these stories has turned what once haunted me into something that honors them. Oakwood goes on without me, but its echoes live in my bones. And despite it all, I am deeply, truly grateful.

At Oakwood, it never failed: I'd walk away from an encounter with a patient—sometimes shaken, sometimes laughing, sometimes both—and think, *"People would never believe this if they weren't here. I should write it down."* But I didn't. Not for years.

When my kids were little and said or did something cute, I used to scribble their funny sayings on scraps of paper and tuck them away. Years later, I found those little pieces of paper, and they brought back the BEST memories.

I never did that with my jail stories—until one day, when a voice in my head nagged: *"Write them. People have no idea what you do in there."*

Once I started, I couldn't stop. I tested my idea on everyone from my doctor to my dentist, my family members, and even my favorite grocery checker, and the reaction was unanimous: *"Yes—tell these stories."* They encouraged me to keep going.

And once I retired, the memories came rushing back. Some were hilarious. Some were heartbreaking. Some were so outrageous they'll stay locked in my private files forever—because if I published them, I might be the one who ends up in court.

When I look back on my 16 years at Oakwood, my heart swells with a bewildering mix of gratitude, grief, awe, and love. I walked through those doors as a nurse, but I left as someone changed—shaped by every inmate who trusted me, every deputy who protected me, every coworker who carried me through shifts that felt impossible. I witnessed horror and resilience, tragedy and humor, cruelty and profound compassion.

Writing forced me to relive everything. From memories that haunted me to memories that honored the people I met. I could picture the cells, hear the keys jangling, remember the sharp mix of adrenaline and compassion that defined each day. The more I wrote, the more my head memories slid into my heart. These weren't just "work stories" anymore; they were evidence of a career I never expected to love, in a place most people never imagine as rewarding.

The public may hear about fights, escapes, riots, deaths, and failures. What they don't hear is that behind those walls are staff who show up every day, balancing toughness with humanity, and sometimes offering an inmate the first scrap of dignity they've had in years. I wanted to make sure someone told *that* side. Oakwood continues without me now, but the echoes of those years—those lives—will stay with me forever, in my heart.

And I'm grateful. To the custody staff who kept me safe, to my coworkers who shared the burden and these amazing experiences—thank you. You made this work possible.

I wanted to take a moment to thank my writing group for your patience and support as I worked on transitioning my writing from a "charting" method to a more readable storytelling style.

I have learned so much from each of you during this process, and I truly appreciate your guidance.

I never thought corrections would be the highlight reel of my career. But it was. The stories will go on without me—but for now, this is where I set down my pen.

Thanks, Oakwood Correctional Facility.

www.ingramcontent.com/pod-product-compliance
Lightning Source LLC
LaVergne TN
LVHW050816061126
851857LV00012B/837
* 9 7 9 8 9 9 7 0 6 7 7 1 7 *